Katja Bredlau-Morich

Kinesiology Taping
FOR HORSES

The Complete Guide to Taping for Equine Health, Fitness, and Performance

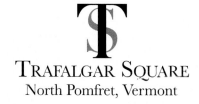

TRAFALGAR SQUARE
North Pomfret, Vermont

To all my equine patients:

You are the reason
I go to work every day.
You are the reason
I am constantly working to improve
myself and my therapeutic skills.
You are the reason
taping applications are constantly
evolving and improving.

First published in the United States of America in 2017 by
Trafalgar Square Books
North Pomfret, Vermont 05053

Revised paperback edition 2024

Originally published in the German language as *Kinesiologisches Pferdetaping*
by Müller Rüschlikon Verlag, Stuttgart

Copyright © 2016 Müller Rüschlikon Verlag, Postfach 103743, 70032 Stuttgart
An imprint of Paul Pietsch Verlage GmbH & Co. KG
Licensee of Bucheli Verlags AG, Baarerstr. 43, CH-6304 Zug

English translation © 2017, 2024 Trafalgar Square Books

Disclaimer of Liability
The authors and publisher shall have neither liability nor responsibility to any
person or entity with respect to any loss or damage caused or alleged to be
caused directly or indirectly by the information contained in this book. While
the book is as accurate as the authors can make it, there may be errors,
omissions, and inaccuracies.

ISBN: 978 1 64601 217 6
Library of Congress Control Number: 2017947931

Photography: Sina Storm: page 11; Caroline Goforth: page 47; all other
photos courtesy of the archives of Katja Bredlau-Morich and Robert Bredlau.
Interior design: R2 | Ravenstein
Cover design: RM Didier
Translation into English: Katja Bredlau-Morich

Printed in the United States of America
10 9 8 7 6 5 4 3 2 1

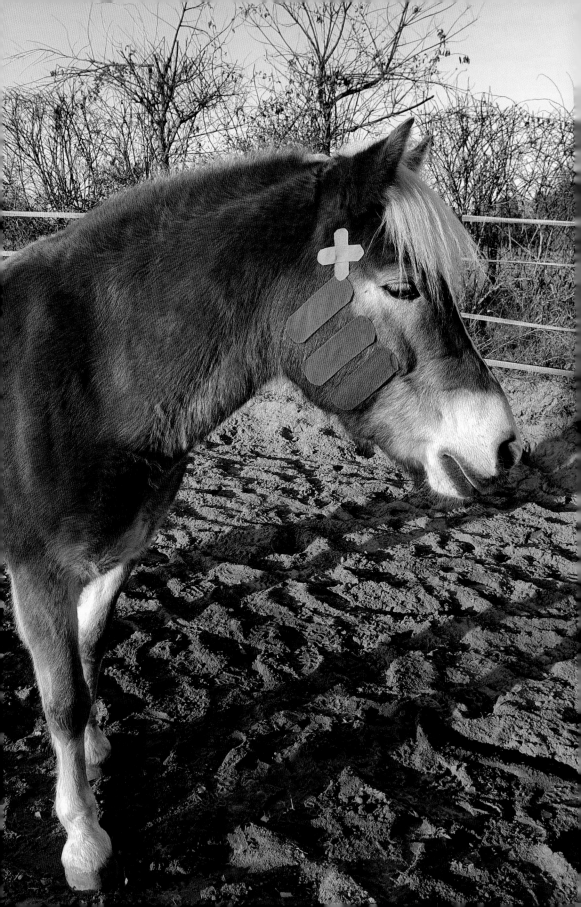

Dear readers,

It is now over seven years since the original German edition of this book was published by Müller Rüschlikon Verlag—and six years since the publication of *Kinesiology Taping for Horses* in the US by Trafalgar Square Books..

A lot has happened in the meantime. From the English translation of this book in 2018, to the German canine version published in 2019 by Kynos Verlag, as well as the English canine version, *Kinesiology Taping for Dogs*, also published by Trafalgar Square Books in 2020.... Taping for animals is attracting more and more interest, and many of our four-legged friends are benefiting from it.

Even though the basic principles of taping remain the same, it's time for a new, completely revised version of this book. All medical and therapeutic treatments are subject to constant change and development. New things are tried out; some of them are discarded, and many of them turn out to be great additions to our understanding of a technique. So here is an update for you: five new chapters, four additional taping applications, and even more case studies, which now immediately follow the taping applications to give you a better overview.

Have fun reading and taping!

Katja Bredlau-Morich

Certified Animal Physiotherapist

Chapter 1

History and Development of Kinesiology Taping

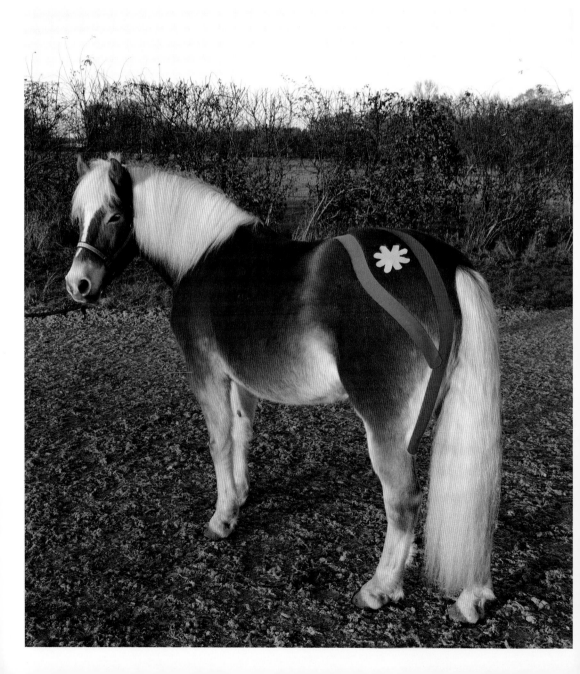

Like so many veterinary treatments, kinesiology taping was not originally developed for horses. It was first designed for human use, and after it proved to be successful there, it was adapted over the years for animals such as horses, cows, dogs, and many more.

The idea for kinesiology taping was developed by Japanese chiropractor Dr. Kenzo Kase in the 1970s, though different sources give different years for the exact date. He had noticed that his chiropractic treatments for his patients often didn't last as long as he would have liked. Thanks to muscle memory and ingrained movement patterns, his patients' problems often came back. Therefore, he was looking for a way to make his own chiropractic treatments last longer, and to support the primary effect of his work.

As mentioned before, this form of tape was developed in the 1970s by Dr. Kenzo Kase. An exact year is difficult to determine, because such a development takes its time. From finding the correct material, the best adhesive, case studies and observation about the effect of the tape on the body, experiences reported by patients and colleagues, up to the serial production; such a thing often can take a long time. That's why you can find various years in the literature.

Taping was not an unknown treatment method at the time, and was used quite frequently—but in a completely different way and style. In the 1970s, therapists worked with "sports tape." This was a very firm and inelastic tape, used to brace and immobilize areas of the body. For example, it was used to immobilize sprained ankles after trauma. Also, bruised or injured fingers were taped to neighboring fingers with it. This sports tape is still used today, and works well in such cases.

But Dr. Kase had something totally different in mind. He was looking for a material that would support tissue and yet allow movement without restricting the patient's range of motion. Based on his experience as a chiropractor, he felt that bracing and immobilization were not always necessarily best for the healing process of soft tissue injuries and problems.

In contrast to a cast, which is quite useful for a broken bone, we now know that a certain amount of controlled, light movement is often better for healing and regeneration of soft tissue injuries. Tendons, ligaments, fasciae, and muscles do benefit from some movement during this period, because it gives the newly formed and regenerated cells the correct impulses, telling them how to align themselves, what they are for, and which way they should grow. With very little or no movement during the rehabilitation phase, disordered cell growth can occur—the cells do not know where to go, where to grow, or what to do.

Based on all these considerations, Dr. Kase developed a stretchable, elastic material that adheres to the surface of the body, and because of its elasticity, can move with tissue and does not restrict a patient's movement.

Depending on the application and technique, kinesiology tape can stimulate or relax muscles, it can loosen fascia, but it can also support joints such as the fetlock joint or vertebrae of the spine and yet there is no restriction of movement in the joint or the muscles. In human practice, kinesiology tape is often even described as a "second layer of skin" because it adapts so perfectly to motion, supporting, stimulating and even improving physiological movement.

In addition to all these considerations, Dr. Kase was looking for a treatment modality that would have a longer-lasting impact on his patients, something that his patients could "take home" with them—that would further

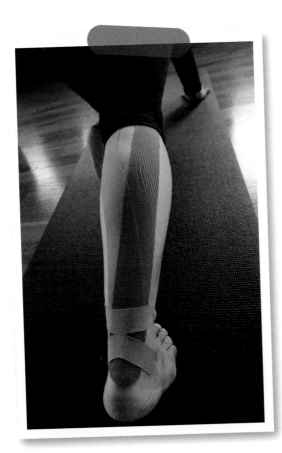

Fig. 1.1: Muscle tape for the calf (*M. gastrocnemius*), combined with a stabilization tape for the Achilles tendon.

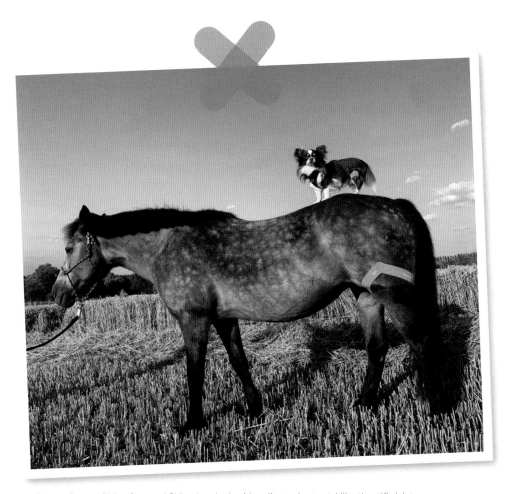

Fig. 1.2: German Riding Pony and Chihuahua, both with a sling taping to stabilize the stifle joint.

promote his chiropractic treatments and "do the work for him," after his patients had left his office. This is possible with kinesiology tape, because the tape can easily remain on the body for several days and do its work. Normal everyday activities are not affected by it: you can wear it at work, you can wear it during sports, you can shower with it—and, and, and....

In both human and veterinary treatment, it is recommended for the tape to stay on for four to five days in the rehabilitation phase, until it comes off by itself, or until you have the feeling that the effect is wearing off. It

can also be used for support during training, and then be removed immediately after the training session.

Kinesiology tape was first seen in public at sporting events in the 1980s. At that time, a few Japanese and Chinese athletes wore these colorful tape strips at sporting competitions. The real breakthrough came in 2008 at the Olympic Games. There, various athletes from different nations used kinesiology tape, wearing it throughout multiple competition events. Four years later, at the Olympic Games in 2012, there was hardly an athlete without kinesiology tape, and many, many athletes from all possible nations were seen wearing it.

From there, it was only a small step to the introduction of kinesiology tape to many doctors' and physical therapists' offices, where it came into daily use. And since it worked so well on humans, the next logical step was taping animals. It is now most commonly used on horses, cows, and dogs. Which probably has to do with their use as riding horses, dairy cattle, or canine sports partners. But many other animals can be treated with tape as well—there are taping applications for cats, guinea pigs, and bunnies, to name a few.

Every horse that is regularly trained in any form performs a certain amount of athletic work, and physical issues and problems can result from this. They should therefore also be treated like athletes. And this does not only mean the top international show horses that perform at their best in major competitions.

Each and every horse can suffer from muscle strains and/or tendon injuries, to just name a few potential problems. Arthritis, malalignment of joints or other physical issues can also cause problems for our four-legged partners. These horses are cared for by veterinarians and therapists (physiotherapists, osteopaths, chiropractors, massage therapists, dorn therapists, etc.) and here the supportive use of kinesiology tape can often be help- and useful. Be it preventive in training or in the aftercare during the rehab phase.

What Does "Kinesiology" Mean?

Before going into detail about kinesiology taping, the "first name" of this tape should be explained in more detail: kinesiology! Where does the term come from? What does it mean? The word "kinesiology" is derived from two Greek words: *kinesis* means **"movement"** and *logia* means **"study"** ("speech," "discussion," or

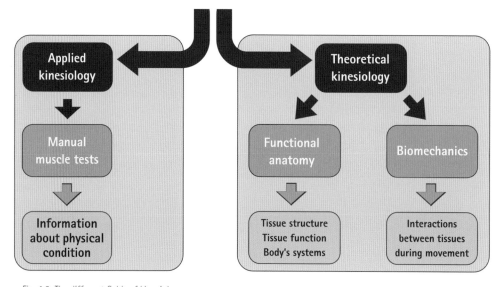

Kinesiology = Study of Movement

Applied kinesiology

→ Manual muscle tests

→ Information about physical condition

Theoretical kinesiology

→ Functional anatomy

→ Tissue structure Tissue function Body's systems

→ Biomechanics

→ Interactions between tissues during movement

Fig. 1.3: The different fields of kinesiology.

"learning" are also accurate translations, depending on context). Thus, kinesiology is the "study of movement." The field of kinesiology can then be further divided into two sub-fields: applied kinesiology and theoretical kinesiology.

Applied kinesiology is an independent method of analysis and treatment. Specific manual muscle tests are performed to check muscle tension. Experienced therapists use these tests to draw conclusions about the functional state of the body.

Theoretical kinesiology, the actual study of movement, deals with the muscles, tendons, ligaments, and bones, as well as their movement, effect, interaction, mutual influence, and dependence on each other. Since everything in the body is interconnected, a great emphasis is placed on the holistic view of the living being. This theory of movement has great influence on training, physical therapy, and rehabilitation for dysfunctional movement.

Theoretical kinesiology can also be divided into two subfields: functional anatomy and biomechanics.

Functional anatomy focuses on the structures of the tissues, musculoskeletal system, and overall organism, as well as the structure and function of each tissue in movement.

Biomechanics focuses on how the above structures interact with each other and how movement affects them.

Definitions: Types of Tape

Everyone who has ever gone to a drugstore to buy kinesiology tape has noticed there are lots of different names and lots of different kinds of tape. So which kind is the kind that is talked about here in the book all the time?

Physio tape: You may hear or see the term "physio tape." This is basically the same as kinesiology tape in terms of material and handling, and is only called by another name by manufacturers in order to highlight its use in physical therapy treatment. This term is now quite widespread in some places; you may see "physio tape" and "kinesiology tape" used side by side, but both describe the same thing. There are even manufacturers who call their tape "kinesiology physio tape."

Sports tape: As described earlier, sports tape is a firm and inelastic material. It braces, supports, and stabilizes the area of the body to which it's applied, and it restricts range of motion.

Dynamic tape: This is a highly elastic tape made of synthetic fiber that is way more stretchable than kinesiology tape. Due to its extreme elasticity, it works primarily through the mechanical recoil forces that are generated when it is applied. With human patients, it's used to correct posture and position. However, this doesn't work well with animal patients, as those strong recoil forces pull on their hair, which they perceive as unpleasant and even painful; it can cause defensive reactions, like kicking, biting, or trying to rid themselves of the dynamic tape.

Chapter 2

Kinesiology Tape—A Special Material

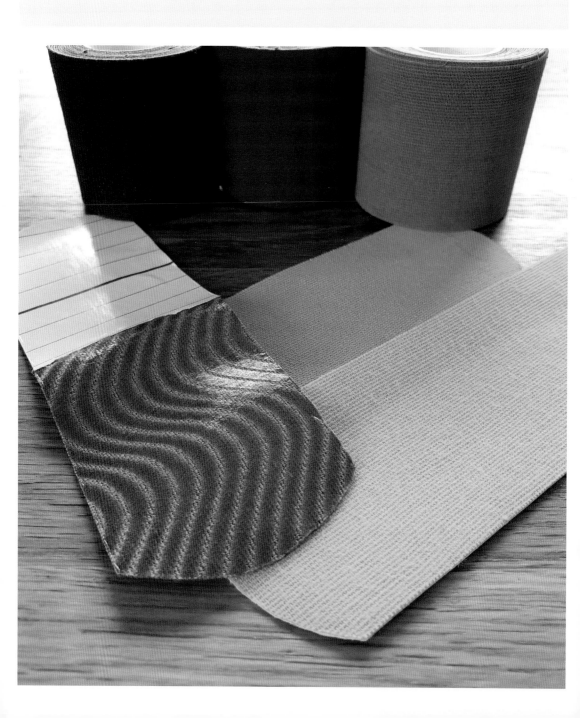

The Material

Kinesiology tape is made of a thin, tightly woven cotton material, similar to a T-shirt or a kitchen towel, interwoven with spandex fibers. These spandex fibers are woven into the tape in the longitudinal direction, so the tape can stretch lengthwise. There isn't any spandex incorporated across the width of the tape—latitudinally—so it doesn't stretch in that direction. This is something you need to keep in mind, especially when taping smaller areas, such as for a scar taping. For these kinds of applications, only small, short tape strips are needed, and you might be tempted to cut across the width of the roll instead of cutting out longitudinal strips. However, as soon as you try to tear the paper on the back, you'll be able to tell that strips cut from across the width of the roll won't stretch; it simply isn't possible without any spandex threads running in that direction through the weave of the tape.

The Elasticity

As previously described, kinesiology tape is interwoven with spandex fibers to make it stretchy and elastic. Like band aids, kinesiology tape is attached to a carrier foil or a paper backing. On this paper, the tape is already pre-stretched by about 10 percent! This pre-stretching is the case with all kinesiology tape, and there are technical reasons for it. If a manufacturer were to try to apply the tape to its paper backing during production without stretching it, it would be likely to wrinkle. So the 10-percent stretch is applied in order for kinesiology tape to lie evenly, wrinkle-free, on its paper backing.

The fact that tape already comes off its paper with this slight pre-stretch should always be kept in mind, especially when taping animals. In a lot of cases this 10-percent pre-stretch is completely sufficient for veterinary taping. In animals, most receptor cells are located in subcutaneous tissue, distributed around the roots of their hair. Therefore, horses, dogs, cats, cows, rabbits, and other animals perceive much more through the fur and the roots of their hair than we humans can perceive through our bare skin.

Depending on the manufacturer, stretchability varies from 140 to 180 percent of the original length of a piece of tape. Different degrees of stretch are clearly visible in kinesiology tapes that have a pattern or name printed on them: the greater the stretch, the more distorted the pattern or lettering.

The Adhesive

On the back, kinesiology tape has a special acrylic adhesive. This adhesive is latex- and

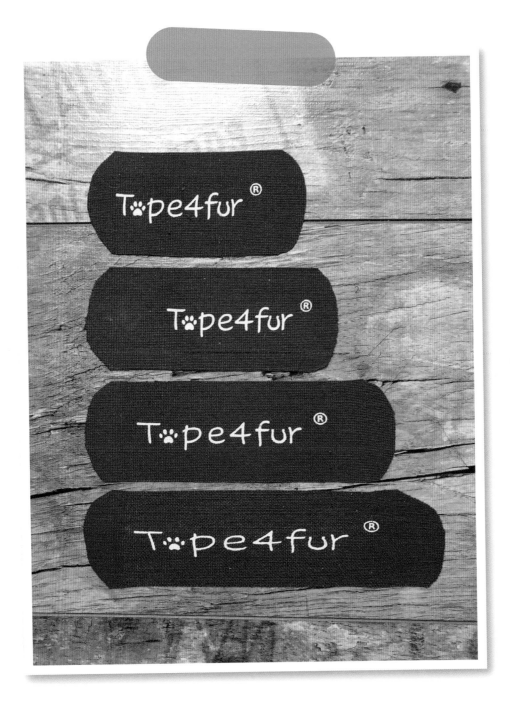

Fig. 2.1: The different degrees of stretch of kinesiology tape. The more stretched the tape is, the more distorted the writing or pattern will be.

Top: No stretch. | Second from top: Mild stretch (10 percent "off-paper" stretch | Second from bottom: Moderate stretch. | Bottom: Strong stretch.

drug-free. If you look at this adhesive layer up close, you can see that it has a wavy pattern, with fine wave-shaped gaps. There is no adhesive in these gaps.

The gaps in between lines of adhesive make kinesiology tape permeable—air and moisture can pass through these spaces, which makes it more comfortable to wear the tape. By contrast, band aids have no gaps in their adhesive, so the skin underneath the adhesive sections doesn't feel so nice after a few days; it often becomes very soft and somewhat paler, and the texture has changed. That gap-free adhesive layer doesn't allow air to pass through, and doesn't allow the skin to "breathe." With kinesiology tape, though, skin can "breathe," thanks to the gaps, and will look perfectly normal even with a tape application that lasts for several days.

There is also a reason for the wave pattern—manufacturers obviously could apply the adhesive, gaps included, in straight lines either lengthwise or crosswise. But during the development of kinesiology tape, testing proved that it adhered better when adhesive was applied in a wave pattern. This may be because bodies don't always move in straight lines, and the wave pattern is able to stick better through movements at all kinds of different angles.

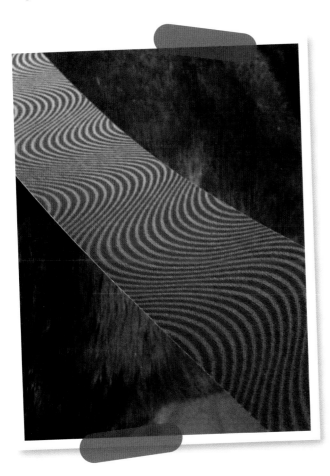

Fig. 2.2: The specific wave pattern of acrylic adhesive on the back of kinesiology tape.

For example, think about the long back muscle. In humans and in horses, this muscle originates at the pelvic bone and then runs parallel to the spine all the way to the occipital bone. This muscle can certainly arch or bend the back forward and backward. But no human or horse moves in a straight line all the time. Picture a horse trying to scratch the side of his belly with his teeth: his back must bend sideways. Or perhaps he lies down to rest, and his back must rotate to the side. A piece of tape applied to the long back muscle must be able to accommodate these movements and compensate for any shear motions or forces that occur. It's been demonstrated that kinesiology tape can best compensate for these issues and stay on through both linear and non-linear movements if the adhesive forms a wave pattern.

The adhesive on kinesiology tape has another special characteristic: it's activated by heat. After applying kinesiology tape to a patient, always rub over it vigorously but carefully; the resulting heat from friction activates the adhesive so it will stick well. There's no specific number of seconds you need to spend rubbing—the only guideline you need is that if your hand gets warm, the tape and the adhesive underneath it have also gotten warm. When the weather is cold, you can also put the horse under a red light for a few minutes. In summer, the sun will do the job just fine.

In Conclusion

The combination of characteristics described above is what makes kinesiology tape so special. The cotton fabric, spandex fibers, and specific adhesive coating make kinesiology tape very similar to skin. This allows it to follow the movements of a patient's body perfectly. The thickness of kinesiology tape is also comparable to the thickness of the uppermost layer of skin. Many human patients report that they don't notice the tape at all after a little while—and horses also tolerate kinesiology tape very well.

Nowadays, there are numerous suppliers for kinesiology tape, and it's available in many different colors. Tapes from one manufacturer are all the same, no matter what color the tape is. Many manufacturers also emphasize that the color makes no difference. However, if you believe in color therapy, it may matter to you which color you use for a particular taping application. More detailed information about this can be found in chapter 4 (page 18).

A question I am often asked is whether all the different brands of kinesiology tape are the same. I always answer unequivocally: Yes and no!

The basics as described above—the cotton fabric, spandex fibers, and acrylic adhesive—are always the same. But there are still differences depending on the manufacturer. For example, the cotton fabric may be thicker or less thick, denser or less dense, and this will affect the tape's stretchability; there can also be very large variations in manufacturers' formulae for the acrylic adhesive, so you may find that some brands of tape stick better for you. Kinesiology tape developed for use on human skin often has too little stretch to be used on horses, which have a massive range of motion, and it also doesn't usually stick well to fur, which means it won't stay in place long enough for equine taping applications to be effective.

In the field of veterinary care, kinesiology tape must perform differently! Veterinary kinesiology tape has to adhere well to fur, not skin. Dirt, dust, and mud also factor in when you're taping four-legged, furry patients, and have to be considered. Human patients rarely roll around in sand or mud with tape applied.

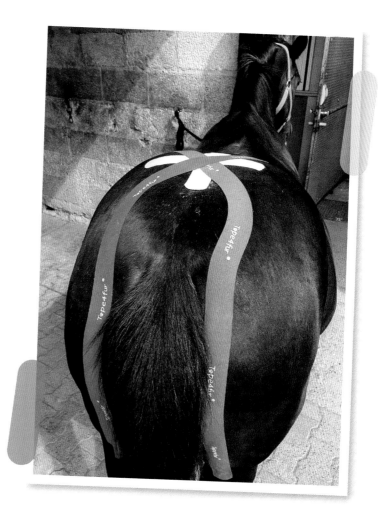

Fig. 2.3: A combination of taping applications: a decompression taping for the SI joints and a muscle taping for the hamstring muscles.

Horses, however, not only enjoy a good roll, but also may stand in the rain in the paddock, or scratch their bodies—and a taping application—with their teeth.

For these reasons, there are some companies focused specifically on manufacturing kinesiology tape for animals. They work with special acrylic adhesives that stick better to fur and can compensate for the difficulties of applying kinesiology tape to animals. A list of some of the most common and most used veterinary kinesiology tapes can be found at the very end of this book.

These special types of tape for animals are usually a bit more expensive, especially compared to the cheap offers for human kinesiology tape that you can sometimes find in discount stores, but the higher price is due to its higher quality. You won't get anywhere if you buy the cheapest tape you can find and then it doesn't adhere properly to the horse's coat—it won't have any effect, and the horse won't get anything out of it. Some people come away saying, "That didn't work at all!" when the problem wasn't the taping application, it was the type of tape they had bought. I strongly recommend that you use tapes that are specially developed and designed for animals and adhere well to fur.

Chapter 3

Kinesiology Tape and Its Effects on Tissue

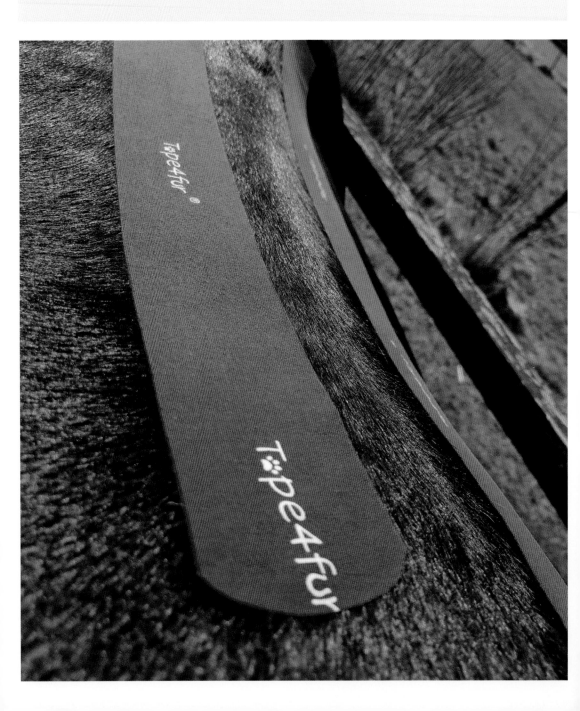

Before we go into more detail about the effects of kinesiology tape, something very important must be said first: Kinesiology taping is a great treatment modality, and you can do a lot of good with it. But it is not a miracle cure that solves all problems by itself!

In my daily work as an animal physiotherapist, I use taping very often. I estimate that about 90 percent of my four-legged patients are sporting colorful taping applications after their treatment sessions.

BUT these taping applications are always preceded by an animal physiotherapy assessment and treatment. Kinesiology taping is a *supportive* modality, intended to bolster, strengthen, and prolong the actual treatment and thus make the primary effect last longer.

Kinesiology taping is quite effective on its own, but it gives the best results when the affected tissue is massaged, loosened, mobilized, activated, stretched, or otherwise treated, depending on an animal physiotherapist's findings, before the tape is applied.

Kinesiology taping is a *supportive* therapeutic modality, meant to complement other forms of therapy (bodywork, massage, stretching, and so on).

General Effect: The "Lifting Effect"

The primary effect of kinesiology tape is based on a simple physical law: anything that is stretched wants to return to its natural unstretched form (a neutral position).

This is true for kinesiology tape as much as for anything else. When kinesiology tape is stretched and applied to skin or animal hair, the stretched material wants to contract again. Since the tape is adhered to the surface of the skin or the ends of the hair, it brings that tissue with it as it tries to contract, pulling on it. The tissue lifts thanks to this pull, because it is being drawn away from the body itself. This is called the **"lifting effect."**

Thanks to this effect, kinesiology tape lifts the skin—or the hair—and this also creates a pull and a lifting effect on the top layer of skin beneath that hair. You can see this clearly in the picture on the next page. When kinesiology tape is applied only to skin, though, the lifting effect is microscopic and cannot be seen. In the picture on the next page, a lot of stretch was intentionally applied to the tape in order to cause extreme contraction and create a very visible lifting effect. **In normal cases, the hair of an animal patient should always be as smooth as possible, and should not stand up like this!**

The lifting effect explained above creates room in the tissue layer underneath the skin. Compressed blood and lymphatic vessels can widen, and blood and lymph fluid can flow more freely. The body's internal waste products can be more easily transported away, and fresh blood and lymph can flow in. This results in better blood circulation, and therefore a better supply of nutrients, minerals, and oxygen for the tissue beneath the taping application. The lifting effect reaches into the next tissue layer, too, and works its way deeper layer by layer.

This means it's possible to influence deeper-rooted problems with kinesiology tape—for example, decompression tapings (star tapings, pain crosses) are often used for horses on their sacroiliac area or for arthritic issues in joints. Arthritis itself is an irreversible process, of course, and that's something kinesiology tape can't change; but it's possible to reduce or even alleviate the accompanying discomfort and pain for an animal. You can often see an improvement in the gait within a few steps after application of a decompression taping.

The lifting effect of kinesiology tape has multiple impacts on tissue

Reducing Pressure

Inflammation, swelling, and painful or tense muscles always come with increased tissue volume. This increase in volume also increases the pressure in the affected area, and on the sensory receptor cells located there.

As described above, kinesiology tape lifts the outermost layers of tissue away from the body,

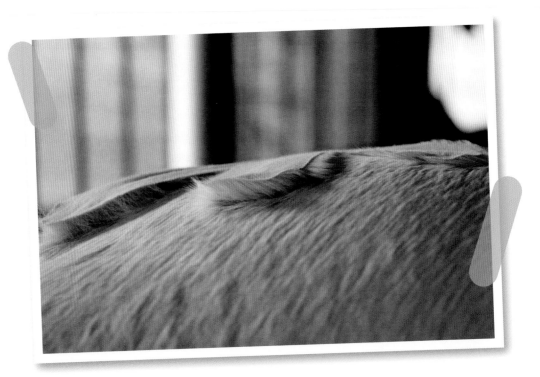

Fig. 3.1: Demonstrating the lifting effect on fur. The middle and leftmost tape strips were applied with **strong stretch**. You can see the equally strong contraction because the fur is sticking up straight. The rightmost taping strip is applied with mild stretch—the amount that should be used in daily practice. Ideally, the hair should lie as flat as possible.

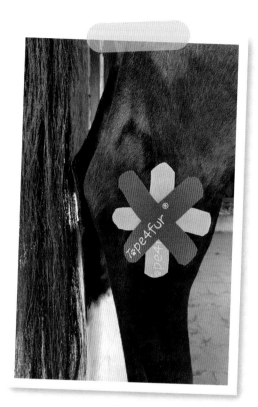

Fig. 3.2: A "pain cross" for arthritis in the hock, with the tape applied to both the medial and lateral sides of the hock.

creating more space. This new space reduces the pressure on inflamed areas, blood and lymph vessels, tense muscles, and sensory receptors.

Relieving Pain

As described above, increased tissue volume causes pressure on sensory receptors—and on pain receptors located in muscle tissue, too, which means inflammation, swelling, and tense muscles cause pain.

As pressure in general decreases on the affected area, pressure on pain receptors also decreases, and the sensation of pain for the patient decreases with it.

Improving Circulation

When there is swelling in joints, extremities, or any other part of the body, or in a case of hematoma, fluid is trapped in the affected tissue. The lifting effect of kinesiology tape creates more space in and around this area, and accumulated fluid such as blood or lymph can drain away more freely, since the blood and lymph vessels in the affected tissue are no longer compressed as tightly. In addition, when tape is applied correctly, the direction in which the tape is contracting physically guides the outflow the right way. Thus, the body's internal waste products (carbon dioxide in the blood, for example) as well as trapped lymph fluid are released. The swelling will be reduced or even eliminated, and blood and lymph circulation improve.

Supporting and Stabilizing Joints

Tense, swollen, or blocked joints also experience an improvement in their function, mobility, and range of motion when pressure on them is reduced by a taping application.

Because kinesiology tape is so similar to skin, as described in chapter 2, it's also possible to support the joints with a special taping technique. For example, the stifle, fetlock joints, or vertebral junctions (see chapter 16, page 124) can be stabilized without restricting their range of motion.

Supporting Muscle Activity

Depending on the application, you can either activate or relax a muscle with the help of kinesiology tape, and that way you can control muscle tone. (This is described in more detail in chapter 10, page 60.) Using the direction in which the tape is applied, and the resulting direction of its recoil, you can support either muscle contraction or muscle relaxation.

In addition, as discussed in the section on circulation, kinesiology taping applications improve blood flow in the taped area, and thus enable better supply of nutrients, minerals, and oxygen to muscle fibers, which has a positive effect on muscle activity.

Improving Body Awareness (Proprioception)

Proprioception is the body's ability to report its own position in relation to its surroundings. If I close my eyes and then move my arm while my eyes are still closed, my brain knows where my arm is and what it is doing—that's my proprioception at work. If I try to touch the tip of my nose with my finger with my eyes closed, it will usually not quite work on the first try. Most of the time, my finger will land close to but next to my nose. Still, my body knows where my arm is, where my nose is, and what my arm has to do so that my finger moves toward my nose—and if I repeat this process, I'll probably touch my nose right on target the next time. The movement will become easier and more purposeful each time I try, and my proprioception improves with each attempt.

Proprioception is based on the signals of specialized sensory cells—proprioceptors—in muscles, fasciae, tendons, and ligaments. The vast majority of proprioceptors are located directly in the subcutaneous fascia and around hair roots. Proprioceptors constantly provide feedback to the brain about the state of the tissue, its tension, and any change in tension.

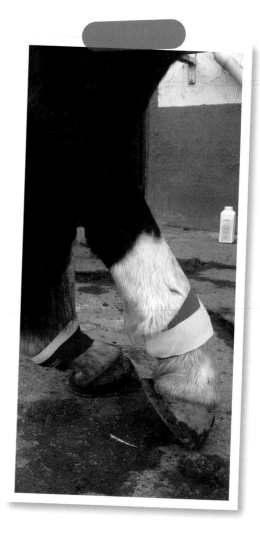

Fig. 3.3: Fetlock support tapings on both legs for an older horse with weak, dropped fetlocks.

Since the superficial fascia and their proprioceptors and mechanoreceptors are located very close to the surface of the skin, it's possible to affect them and improve body perception with the help of kinesiology tape.

Example: Improvement of Body Awareness

During one of my taping courses, I had a "model horse" that always dragged her toes when she was maneuvering her forehand. There was no reason for it; her muscles, tendons, and joints were all fine. After the application of a proprioception taping, the owner reported that same evening that the horse not only no longer dragged her toes, but no longer bumped the small pole that lay on the ground between her stall and the paddock.

Every taping application has an impact on body awareness, because the proprioceptors are so close to the surface of the skin—but there are also specific taping techniques that can be used to target proprioception in particular. You can find out more about this in chapter 20.

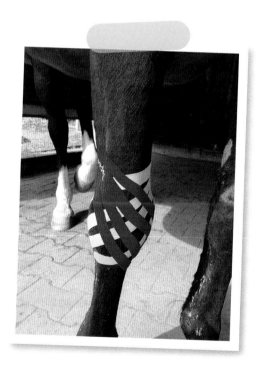

Fig. 3.4: A proprioception taping at the carpal joint to help activate the front leg.

Chapter 4

Colors and Their Significance

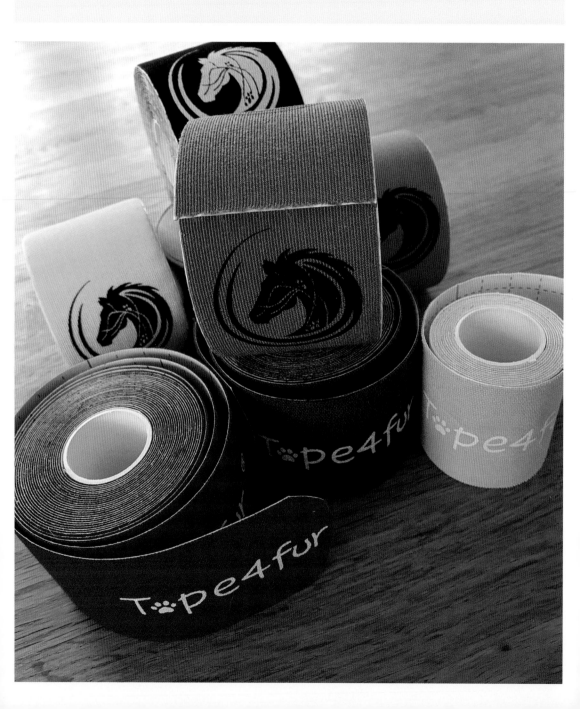

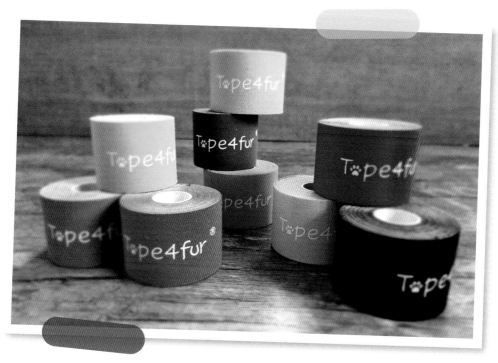

Fig. 4.1: Kinesiology tape is available in many different colors.

Kinesiology tapes are now offered by many different manufacturers, and each manufacturer has their own selection of colors.

There are no differences between different colors in the same brand in terms of how the tape is made, so all colors are equally effective. Within any given brand, all of the actual kinesiology tape will be identical: it will use the same cotton fabric with the same thickness and the same adhesive formula, and the adhesive will be put on every color of tape the same way. The sole difference is which color of dye is applied to the cotton fabric.

Why, then, is kinesiology tape produced in different colors? Manufacturers don't attribute any particular effects to different colors—for them, it's simply a matter of marketing. Customers feel catered to when they have

choices; being able to pick out a color you like is a more enjoyable shopping experience than looking at a shelf of identical off-white rolls of kinesiology tape.

Nevertheless, many animal therapists, especially holistic therapists, believe that color does make a difference, and that different colors have different effects in treatment.

In ancient times, healers experimented with colors and included them in holistic medical treatments. The sick were covered with colored pastes, or wrapped in colored cloths. Johann Wolfgang von Goethe, the nineteenth-century German writer, poet, and natural philosopher, also discussed colors and their effects in his work. Color therapy exists today as a pseudoscientific supportive treatment modality.

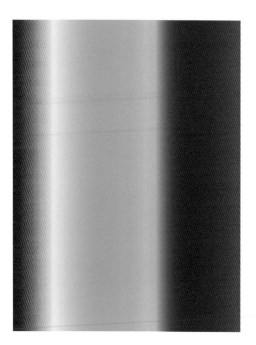

Fig. 4.2: The color spectrum, from infrared to ultraviolet.

In the context of human vision, there is a clearly defined color spectrum that runs from infrared to ultraviolet. Each color corresponds to a specific wavelength of light with a defined nanometer range; for example, light at 450 nm looks blue to human eyes, and light at 710 nm looks red. In addition, each color also corresponds to a frequency in the terahertz range: a frequency of 650 THz looks blue, for example, and 420 THz looks red.

Since different colors reflect and absorb different frequencies of light, in a certain sense it's not impossible that applying coverings of different colors to certain areas of the body might make a measurable difference.

The Effect of Color in Kinesiology Taping

Early in my kinesiology taping career, I had not yet given any thought to color theory or the possible effects of colors. During treatment of a horse with severe back tension, I chose to use red tape, just because I liked the color. The application adhered well to the horse, and his back pain decreased significantly.

On a follow-up treatment for the same horse, I happened to grab blue tape instead. To my surprise, when I tried to use it, the blue tape did not stick at all. Even after repeated, thorough cleaning of the horse's coat, it just didn't stick. Trying a different roll of blue tape gave me the same result. Then I went back to the red tape—which was from the same manufacturer as the blue tape—and this time, the application adhered perfectly.

According to color theory, blue has a cooling effect and red has a warming effect. Muscular tension is treated with heating pads, red light, and fango (a mud mixture that is heated before application) in humans; I decided perhaps the tense back muscle of this horse also wanted some warming red tape, and not cooling blue tape.

Nowadays, I carry up to 8 colors with me to choose from (red, yellow, green, dark and light blue, pink, orange, purple, and black) and usually ask the owners of my four-legged patients which color they would like for their animal. Many horse owners don't care about the color and leave the choice up to me. But in many cases, the owners choose the color that I would have chosen based on color therapy.

Red

Red is one of the three primary colors in color theory, also called a basic color. This means that it is not created by mixing other colors. According to color theory, red has a dynamic, invigorating, stimulating effect, and increases energy, vitality, blood circulation, and activity; it has a positive effect on the sensory nervous system and metabolism, and is warming.

Wavelength: 640–780 nm
Frequency: 470–380 THz

Yellow

Yellow is also one of the three primary colors. In color theory, yellow has a stimulating and warming effect, but not quite as much as red; it gathers and harmonizes energy, and has a positive effect on glands and the lymphatic system. The color yellow is supposed to promote the function of internal organs, such as the liver, spleen, gallbladder, stomach, and intestines.

Wavelength: 570–600 nm
Frequency: 530–500 THz

Blue

Blue is the third primary color. According to color theory, it has a relaxing and calming effect, and is cooling; it causes physical relaxation and stress reduction, and lowers blood pressure. Due to its attributed cooling and antiseptic effect, therapists who believe in color theory often use it in cases of fever, inflammation, or sunburn.

Wavelength: 430–490 nm
Frequency: 700–610 THz

Pink

Pink is a secondary color, obviously closely related to red. Depending on the brightness of its hue, pink is said to have a gentle or soothing effect, and lead to inner peace and serenity or lighten mood. As with red, the color pink is attributed an energizing effect.

Pink is not included in the classic color spectrum; scientifically, it is essentially an illusion created by the human brain when we perceive a mixture of red and purple light.

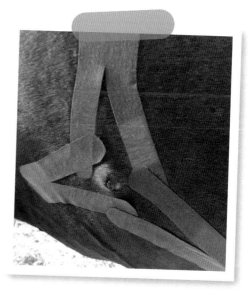

Fig. 4.3: A blue hematoma taping for a very swollen insect bite.

Green

Green is considered a secondary color in color theory, created by mixing the primary colors yellow and blue (this is not scientifically accurate when it comes to colors of light, however). It is supposed to have the greatest healing, regenerating, and relaxing effect of any color, and is considered balancing, harmonizing, neutralizing, and calming; it is often referred to as "the healing color" by therapists who believe in color theory.

Wavelength: 490–570 nm
Frequency: 610-530 THz

Purple

Purple is also considered a secondary color in color theory, created by mixing the primary colors red and blue. Therapists who believe in color theory disagree about its effects, which may be because it combines colors of ostensibly opposing natures (warming red and cooling blue). Depending on the shade, it may be used to harmonize and calm, but also to give energy, and supposedly promotes concentration.

Wavelength: 380–430 nm
Frequency: 790–700 THz

Orange

Orange is the third secondary color in color theory, considered a mixture of red and yellow (though, again, this reflects usage of dyes and pigments and not the science of light), and is thought of as combining their effects. It is used by therapists who believe in color theory as a strength-giver after physical or mental exhaustion, and represents vital strength and activity. Because of its comprehensive stimulat-

ing effect, orange is also used in color therapy to strengthen the immune system and activate the body's defenses. It is supposed to have an uplifting, invigorating, positive, and in every way health-promoting effect, and is even attributed the ability to encourage appetite and stimulate digestion.

Wavelength: 585–650 nm
Frequency: 510–460 THz

Black

Within the spectrum of visible light, there is no wavelength or frequency corresponding to black; black is **not a color of light**, but a state of the eye! If no light is reflected to the eye by a surface, that surface appears black.

According to color therapy, similarly, black is the absence of color; it is believed to drain energy and therefore should never be used in states of exhaustion.

Since it is by definition not a color, black cannot be assigned a specific wavelength or frequency.

I use black kinesiology tape mostly to create anchors to secure an actual taping application. For me, it typically has no function at all except to help keep applications of other colors in place.

Occasionally, however, I do use black tape more extensively, when I am treating an animal with a very high energy level (not too high, but high). I apply black kinesiology tape to nervous, fidgety, overexcited, and overstimulated animals in order to "anchor" them energetically, and "slow them down"!

Whether you believe in color theory or not, and whether you want to incorporate color selection into your treatment or not, is, of course, up to you. I know colleagues, especially in the field of holistic animal treatment, who believe color selection is crucial to the success of a taping application. But I also know colleagues for whom tape color plays no role at all—who, for example, tape every application using pink, because it is their favorite color and looks pretty. Everyone must decide how to use or not use color for themselves. Personally, I usually go by my gut feeling; when I do a muscle taping on a highly tense muscle, I almost always find myself using red tape. According to color theory, red will warm the muscle, and this warmth will provide it with energy, which the muscle needs for regeneration and relaxation. When I do a tendon taping, on the other hand, I usually use blue, since blue is believed to have a cooling effect, and tendons tend to prefer it cool.

Fig. 4.4: Most manufacturers of kinesiology tape make all kinds of colors for the customer to choose from.

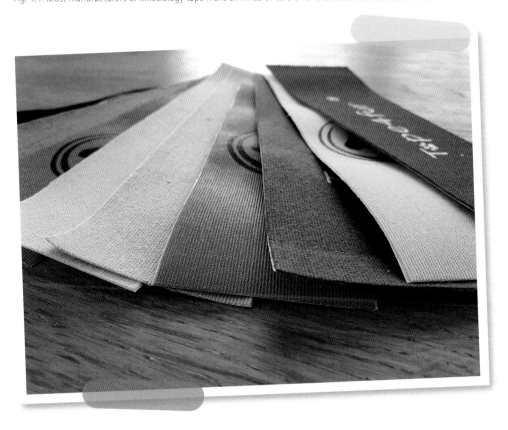

Chapter 5

Indications for Equine Kinesiology Taping

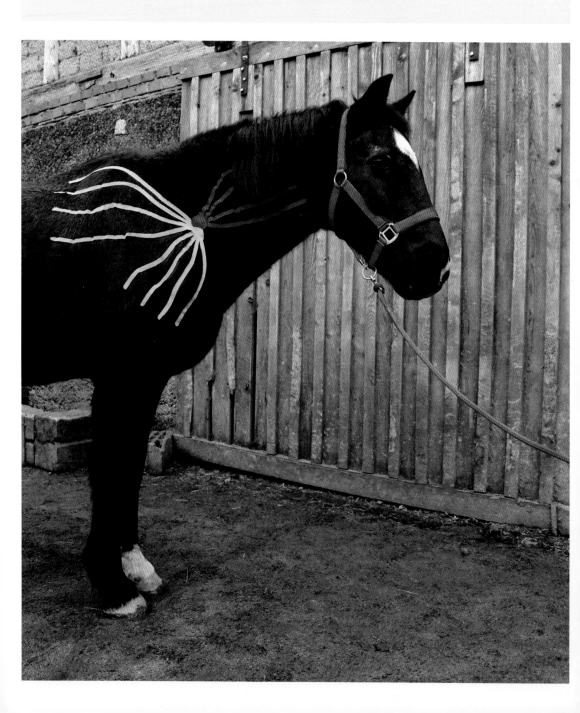

In addition to my explanation of the effects of kinesiology tape in chapter 3, you should also know in which cases and with which conditions kinesiology tape should be used.

In General

Kinesiology tape is generally very helpful in cases of fatigue after hard work, training, or exercise, such as horse show days with several tests. Due to its ability to promote circulation, it supports the regeneration and reinvigoration of muscles after increased work and heavy stress, among other things.

Since applying kinesiology tape can affect proprioceptors, issues involving body aware-ness and balance can also be addressed. Kinesiology tape's effect on circulation also means it can shorten rehabilitation times. Because it behaves so much like skin, it adds an extra "layer" to the tissue, so it can increase stability, depending on the taping application.

Kinesiology tape can also be used preventa-tively. For example, tendon tapes can be used in advance of increased training to give tissue more support and prevent tendon damage. Similarly, you can tape certain muscle areas in advance of specific kinds of training in order to increase stimulation of those areas during riding.

Muscle Issues

Depending on the amount of exercise the horse is getting—or a lack thereof—his musculature may be *hypertonic* or *hypotonic*, *atrophic* or *hypertrophic*. (For definitions, see chapter 9, page 54.) Muscles may also be in a state of *rigidity* or *spasm*. With the help of kinesiology tape and its "lifting effect," the blood vessels supplying a muscle or group of muscles can be widened again; this means the musculature is better supplied with blood and can recover faster. Depending on the direction in which a muscle taping is applied, and the resulting direction of recoil of the tape, hypertonic muscles can be relaxed, or hypotonic muscles can be stimulated and activated. For more specifics, see chapter 10 (page 60).

Fascia Issues

Muscular tension is not the only kind of tension that can be relieved and regulated with kinesiology tape—tension in the superficial fascia can also be addressed with a taping application. The fascia surrounds muscles as well as organs, and if it gets tight and re-stricted, it can stick together, disrupting the function of the underlying tissue. Special taping techniques are used to address the superficial fascia that is closest to the surface of the skin. These fascia tapings help reorganize the fascia and restore its mobility. For more specifics, see chapter 11 (page 92).

Arthritis and Arthrosis

Osteoarthritis is unfortunately a very common problem in horses today. Growth disorders (genetically determined), incorrect posture and stress on the bones (acquired), or even overloading of the skeletal system can lead to degenerative degradation and problems for bones and joints. Even the best kinesiology tape cannot reverse osteoarthritis itself, but it can alleviate the accompanying symptoms. For example, a muscle taping can stimulate the muscles surrounding an affected osteoarthritic area, or a decompression taping can take the pressure off the tissue or joint and thus relieve pain.

Swelling

If a horse has swollen legs—for example, after operations or injuries, or due to a bruise or lymph congestion—kinesiology tape can be used to stimulate circulation, which can reduce or even eliminate swelling. The lifting effect of the tape, as well as the direction of recoil through it, can be harnessed to stimulate and support drainage of fluids and metabolic waste products. For more specifics, see chapters 14 and 15 (page 108 and page 118 respectively).

Joint Instability

By using certain application techniques to maintain tension and suppress the instant recoil of the tape, kinesiology taping applications can support the stability of joints without restricting their range of motion. The tape covers the joint like a second skin, and gives it additional support without compressing it. This can be very helpful in cases of, for example, instabilities in the joints of the spine, as well as

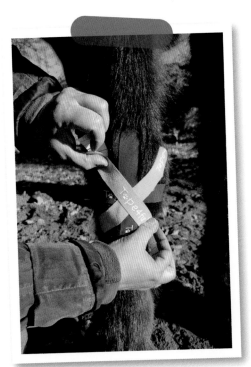

Fig. 5.1: Decompression taping on a carpal joint with osteoarthritis.

in the extremities. For more specifics, see chapter 13 (page 98).

Trigger Points

The decompressing effect of the kinesiology tape can be used to relieve localized hardened areas in the musculature, and possibly even to release them, or to encourage their release in combination with other treatments. All taping applications have a decompressing effect, but a greater impact can be achieved with deliberate use of spacing and by overlaying multiple strips of tape over a particular point. For more specifics, see chapter 12 (page 90).

Scar Tissue

Scar tissue is often inelastic and rigid; these limitations can be addressed by using the recoil of kinesiology tape to stimulate this tissue to give way. The lifting effect of kinesiology taping also increases blood flow, and therefore the supply of nutrients and oxygen, to the area around a taped scar. However, this kind of taping treatment is often a rather lengthy process; it takes time for scar tissue to become supple and mobile again. Therefore, especially when treating older scars, it's important to apply a scar taping multiple times. For more specifics, see chapter 17 (page 130).

Tendon Injuries, Strains, and Tears in the Extremities

Tendon damage and injuries are unfortunately a very common problem with our four-legged partners. And it isn't just excessive riding that can cause this. Romping around in the paddock with other horses can also lead to overstretching and strains, and even tendon ruptures. Here, too, kinesiology tape can improve blood circulation, which encourages recovery, and the tape's direction of recoil can help relieve strain on the affected tendon after overstretching. Increased circulation means the damaged tissue is supplied with more oxygen and nutrients, which helps the damaged tendon heal.

For animals prone to tendon problems or horses with dropped fetlocks, tendon taping is also recommended as a preventative treatment during training. For more specifics, see chapter 16 (page 124).

Pain

In general, any taping application will provide some degree of pain relief, due to the "lifting effect"—when tissue is less compressed, metabolic waste products drain from it more easily, and pressure on pain receptors is reduced. This is also why decompression tapings specifically have the greatest pain-relieving effect; they are not nicknamed the "pain cross" for nothing. For more specifics, see chapter 12 (page 90).

Limited Body Awareness

Many horses have a preferred diagonal, which they load more than the other—for example, their right forefoot and their left hind. This is not unusual; we humans are right- or left-handed, and horses are essentially right-to-left- or left-to-right-diagonal-legged. However, in some cases, this uneven loading gets out of hand, and various stresses and strains along these diagonals can occur. In these cases, a proprioception taping helps direct the horse's body awareness back to his other diagonal, or to another limb, in order to restore balance in his body. For more specifics, see chapter 20 (page 148).

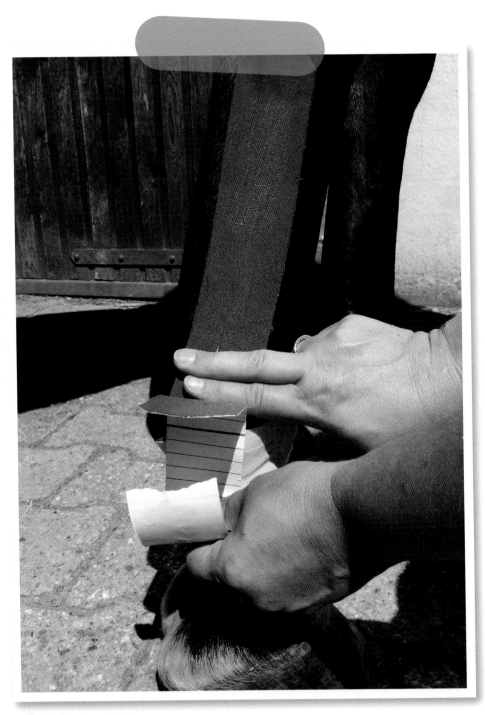

Fig. 5.2: A tendon taping for the deep digital flexor tendon.

Supplementing Training

As mentioned a few times previously, certain taping applications can also be used preventatively, or to augment the effects of training. Muscle tapings, for example, can target specific muscles during training; tendon tapings can support weak, vulnerable tendons during riding.

Some polo teams I have worked with, for example, apply simple tendon tapings during polo training sessions (covering them with polo wraps while practicing), and have experienced significantly less recurring tendon damage in their polo ponies.

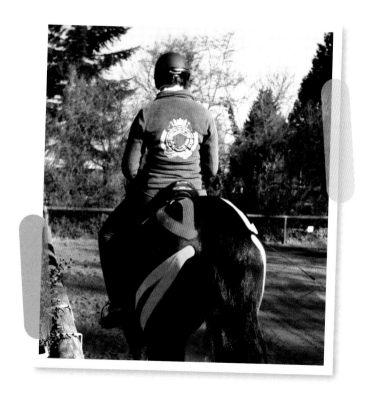

Fig. 5.3: Muscle taping of the gluteal and hamstring muscles during riding, to support these muscles and encourage hind leg activity.

Chapter 6

Contraindications for Equine Kinesiology Taping

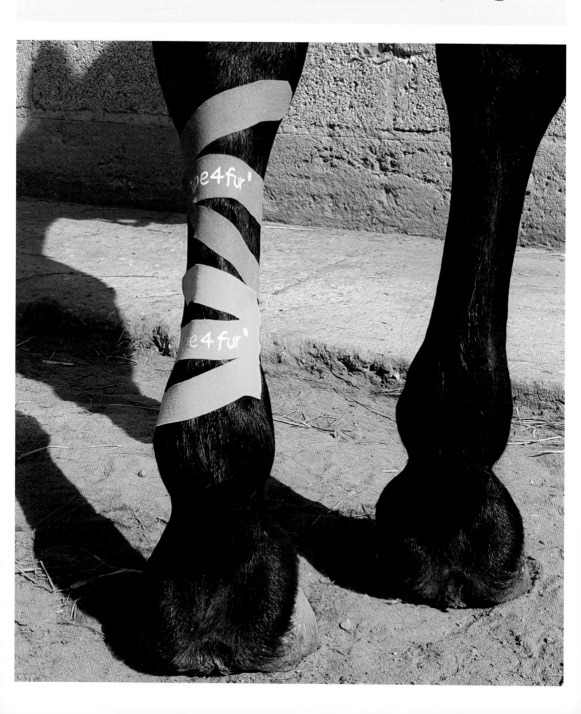

As with almost all physiotherapeutic treatment methods for horses, there are of course some clinical symptoms and situations for which kinesiology taping is not advisable, and you should refrain from applying tape.

Skin Diseases

In cases involving skin diseases, including fungal issues, avoid applying kinesiology tape. While the tape might be able to help the tissue underneath the affected skin, the risk of spreading the disease or fungus farther is too high. The situation might also continue to deteriorate beneath the tape, and you would not be able to see or treat this acceleration until the tape was removed, leaving the situation in worse shape than when treatment began. In addition, you (or the therapist undertaking the taping) might come into contact with fungal spores or other pathogens when you are touching the horse's skin and hair with your hands, or with the tape—which means you might spread the disease or fungus to other parts of the horse's body, or to other patients. Fungal spores are everywhere, but there is no need for us to encourage their distribution. Hands and scissors should be washed thoroughly after every taping application; but tape rolls cannot be washed, and since you have to hold the roll directly against your four-legged patient and his coat to measure out the correct length of tape, there is no way for you to avoid having the tape roll touch the horse.

Open Wounds

Kinesiology taping should also be avoided in areas where the horse has one or more open wounds. Taping over an open wound is impossible in any case, because kinesiology tape will not stick to wet or bloody areas. However, taping too close to a wound is also a bad idea, and could negatively impact healing. As mentioned previously, taping applications stimulate blood flow—which could cause excessive scarring or "proud flesh." As soon as a wound has fully closed, scabs have fallen off on their own, and any stitches have been removed, you can certainly consider applying a treatment like a scar taping.

If there is swelling around an open wound, you can apply a hematoma taping around the general area of the injury, but not directly over it!

Fever

Most physiotherapeutic treatment modalities are aimed at stimulating circulation, and thus blood flow. This also applies to kinesiology taping. When a horse presents with fever, however, his body needs all its energy for its own immune defense—you should therefore refrain from physiotherapeutic treatment and taping. Instead, contact your veterinarian. After successful treatment, when the elevation in the horse's temperature has subsided, you can apply physiotherapeutic treatment or taping.

Localized Infections

Unfortunately, horses can sometimes be prone to lymphangitis: a small scratch, a tiny injury, and suddenly the whole leg is swollen, and possibly even inflamed and hot. In cases like these, a lymph taping could potentially be useful to drain the stocked-up fluid. However, for as long as a swollen area remains percepti-bly hot because of an infection, **DO NOT** apply tape to that area! Because kinesiology taping applications increase circulation, using them on an infected area risks spreading the infection throughout the body and making the situation

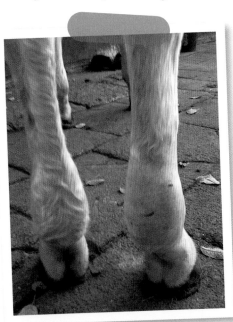

Fig. 6.1: Lymphangitis around the fetlock of the right hind leg.

even worse. However, if an infection is completely gone and only residual swelling remains, taping the area with a lymphatic tape can help.

Pregnancy

When it comes to human therapeutic care, pregnant people now sometimes have kinesiology tape applied to support their stretched and strained connective tissue. But people can also remove the kinesiology tape themselves immediately if they notice that it does not do them any good or they do not feel comfortable with it. This is only partially possible with horses, and therefore kinesiology tape should not be used on pregnant mares. You can never predict exactly what may cause contractions or premature labor; avoid any risk for mare and foal, and refrain from taping a mare in the area of the trunk, belly, and abdomen during pregnancy.

Colic

Colic is clearly a case for the vet! Physiothera-peutic treatments and taping are both very much out of place in this case. It's only natural to feel a need to help your horse in any way you can and do something to ease his pain, but the symptoms he is experiencing should not be covered up by a pain-relieving taping applica-tion. The vet won't thank you if crucial symptoms are masked and accurate diagnosis becomes difficult or impossible—and the horse probably won't either, if he does end up in the hospital. Even if that were not true, a taping would be inadvisable; most horses will not tolerate treatment or taping around the belly very well when in severe, acute pain.

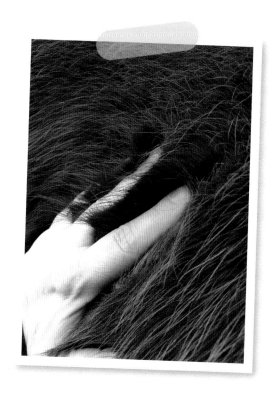

Fig. 6.2: A very long winter coat can be difficult to tape, and given the length of this coat, it is difficult to say how much of the lifting effect of the kinesiology tape actually reaches the skin and its receptors, which limits how effective the tape can be.

Malignant Tumors

As described several times previously, kinesiology tape increases circulation in the area where it is applied. This is not a good thing when malignant tumors are involved; they may grow or spread even farther through the body. If a patient is known to have malignant tumors, this is a definite contraindication!

Allergy or Hypersensitivity

I have never seen or experienced it myself in over 10 years of practice—but it is possible, in unusual cases, for horses to have an allergic reaction to kinesiology tape, or to the acrylic adhesive. In this case, please remove the kinesiology tape from the horse's coat immediately and wash the affected area with plenty of warm water.

Long or Thick Coat

The shorter the horse's coat, the more effective a taping application will be. High-quality tapes that have been developed specifically for use on animals will usually adhere to longer fur without any problems. But imagine, for example, an Icelandic horse in winter, living outside, with a super-long, plushy-thick coat. It is difficult to say how much of the lifting effect would actually reach the skin in this case, given the length of the hair and extreme thickness of the coat. A Warmblood with an average winter coat can usually be taped without an issue. In the case of an Icelandic horse, however, I usually do not do any taping in winter.

Chapter 7

Preparing the Horse and His Coat

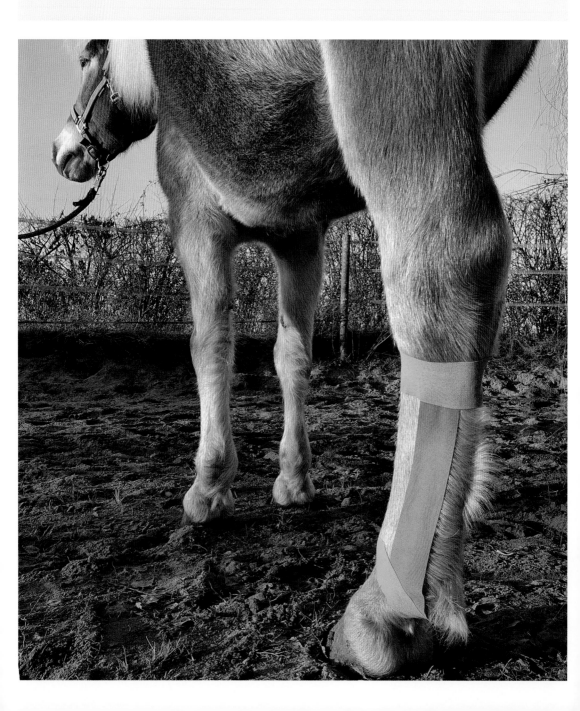

In General

The most important factor when you are preparing to apply kinesiology tape is whether the horse is clean. Kinesiology tape does not stick very well if there is dirt and dust between the adhesive and the horse's coat. So the horse should be thoroughly bathed before his taping session begins.

However, he needs to be washed far enough in advance of the taping that he also has time to dry—kinesiology tape does not stick to wet hair at all. If the horse's owner thinks the horse needs a bath, they should do it the day before the treatment in order to ensure the horse is completely dry again for his appoint-

ment. Even when a horse has been washed with time to spare, days with very high humidity or heavy rain can make applying tape to hair difficult.

You should also refrain from using fly and shine sprays on areas that will be taped. These sprays smooth the structure of the coat, which will make it harder for the kinesiology tape to adhere to areas where they are applied. This effect is immediately noticeable; the tape will just roll right off the hair. However, it is perfectly fine to apply fly spray after tape is applied, including over the taped area.

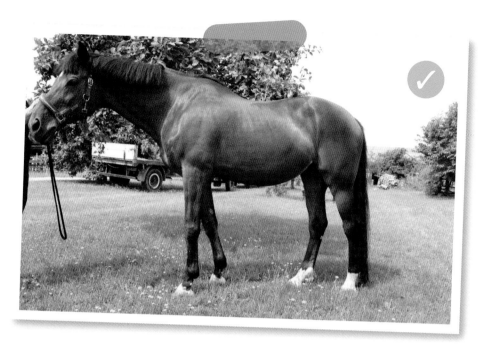

Fig. 7.1: The horse should be dry and clean to ensure the kinesiology tape will stick well.

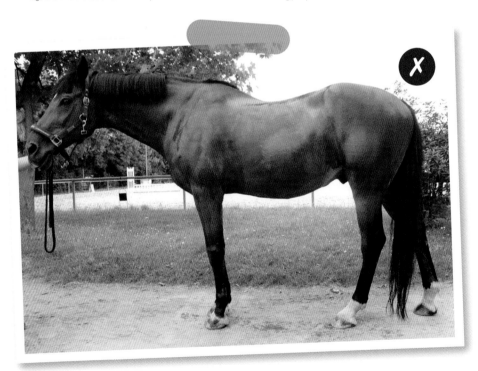

Fig. 7.2: Tape will not adhere to wet hair! In this case, an application is simply not possible.

Tips and Tricks to Improve Adhesion

Clipping the Horse

I am often asked whether a horse should be clipped before his taping session. You certainly can clip in advance, but you don't have to. So far, I have never felt like I had to stop at the beginning of a taping and ask for a horse to be clipped before I could proceed. Tapes that have been developed specifically for use on animals stick very well, even when applied to an average horse's winter coat. The exceptions are Shetland or Icelandic Ponies with extremely thick, long winter coats. Kinesiology tape will adhere to a long coat, but it is hard to say how much of the tape's effect would still reach the skin and its receptors, given the length and thickness of the hair. This kind of coat is, in effect, a contraindication, as already described in chapter 6. Clipping an Icelandic Pony in winter just for the sake of a taping session is counterproductive—after all, he has his thick, long winter coat for a reason!

By contrast, I *have* experienced the problem of tape not sticking to the extremely short hair of a freshly clipped horse. I arrived at the barn right after the horse's clipping session, and his hair was so short that it did not lie smoothly against his body, but rather stood up like a buzzcut, with the hair forming hedgehog-like bristles. The tape could not stick to the ends of the hair alone—it was like trying to apply a band-aid to a hairbrush.

So I made another appointment for the horse 14 days later; his coat had grown back a bit by then, and taping was not a problem anymore.

Spray Adhesive

There are some horses that are very difficult to tape, because they simply have naturally greasier skin and hair than most. Certain manufacturers have developed special spray adhesives that are useful for horses like these. Simply use the spray adhesive on the area to be taped before applying the tape to the horse, and it will stick better. This problem of greasier skin and hair is relatively common in Nordic breeds such as Shetland, Icelandic, or Norwegian Ponies—presumably because in nature, the extra coating helped keep their ancestors warmer in cold weather. This also sometimes occurs in horses that are fed oils as a supplement with their food.

Overall, I am not an advocate of spray adhesives for horses. I bought a bottle of spray adhesive at the beginning of my "taping career," and years later I found it still sealed in the trunk of my car. The expiration date had long since passed. I simply dislike applying spray adhesive to a healthy and intact coat—unlike the adhesive on the reverse side of the kinesiology tape, which only adheres to the surface of the coat, spray adhesive penetrates deeper into the structure of the hair, potentially clogging it.

I also suspect that applying tape to a coat using spray adhesive reduces the recoil in the tape and severely compromises the minimal shear forces between the tape and the hair roots and proprioceptors, which is extremely important for improving body awareness. So I think spray adhesive can actually be counterproductive.

Baby Powder

To optimize the stickiness of my tape when I need to, I prefer to use conventional baby powder instead of spray adhesive. Baby powder was developed to keep babies' bottoms dry in their diapers, and it will do the same with a horse's hair.

If I notice that my tape is not sticking well, due to moisture or greasiness in the horse's hair, I remove the application. Then I take regular baby powder, spread it over the area to be taped, and rub it in lightly. After giving it a few minutes to absorb the moisture or grease, I remove it again with a microfiber cloth. This step must be done very thoroughly; tf too much baby powder remains in the hair, the tape will stick to the powder and not to the hair, and it won't stick any better than it did before! Microfiber cloths are perfect for this purpose, as they really attract dust—and also baby powder. When the baby powder is completely gone and the horse's coat is dry and free of grease, nothing stands in the way of the taping application.

One Last Word

In very rare cases, you sometimes cannot get the tape to stick no matter what tricks you try. My 10 years and counting of taping experience have taught me there is usually a reason why kinesiology tape does not want to stick to a horse. In my opinion, this is a sign that the body does not want or need the tape! In these rare cases, you should not bother the horse with continued attempts to tape him.

Can the Horse Be Ridden While the Kinesiology Tape Is in Place?

Again and again, horse owners stand next to me while I tape their horses and ask me: "Can I ride my horse now? Do I need to pay special attention to anything? Does my horse need stall rest because of the tape?"

Well, what really matters here is why the horse needs treatment and taping in the first place! A horse that is on stall rest due to tendon damage, diagnosed by a veterinarian, needs to stay on rest when he has a tendon tape in place—not because of the taping application, but because of the underlying condition the taping application is helping to treat.

By contrast, there are certain taping applications—for example, specific muscle tapes—that are applied specifically in order to support and augment the effects of training. As long as there are no other conditions at play that restrict this training, the horse can and should be ridden with the tape applied.

In general, as long as the horse is allowed to move as he usually does without the tape, he is allowed to do so once the tape is on. Similarly, when we humans are taped, we move around as usual, unless there is a specific reason we should abide by a movement restriction.

For me, there is one category of exceptions to this rule: taping of the long back muscle and other applications that go on the back of the horse, under the saddle. As described in chapter 3, kinesiology tape works through the lifting effect. If I have taped the long back muscle or, for example, applied a fascia tape for the thoraco-lumbar back fascia, and then a saddle and a rider are placed on top of the taping application, that physical load will counteract the lifting effect completely. With taping applications that are positioned on the horse's back, I recommend a break from riding of about 3–4 days; the kinesiology tape should be removed before the saddle and rider get to go back on the horse again.

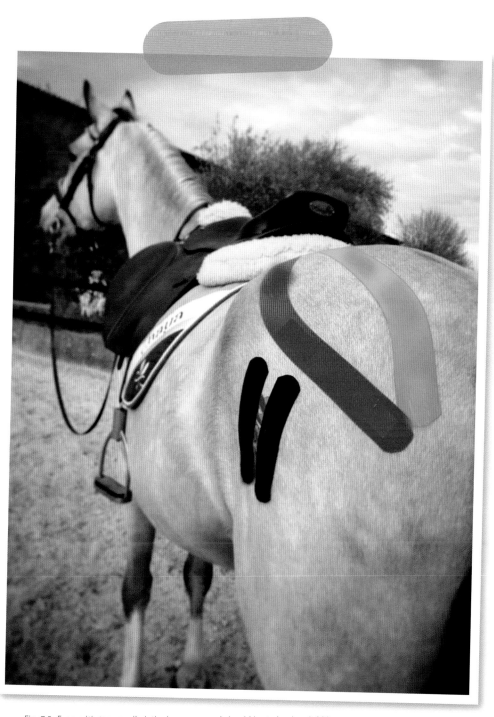

Fig. 7.3: Even with tape applied, the horse can and should be trained and ridden.

Chapter 8

Preparing and Handling
Kinesiology Tape

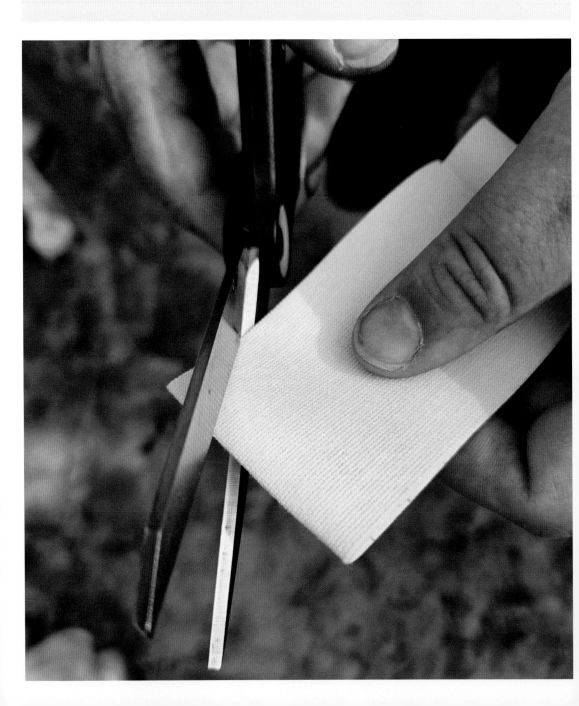

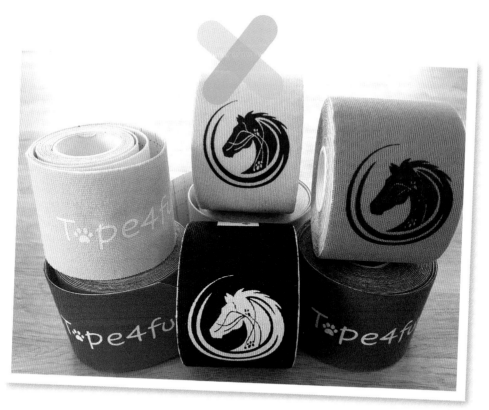

Fig. 8.1: Kinesiology tapes from different brands in multiple widths and colors.

Tape Selection

Today, kinesiology tape is available from many different suppliers, and some tapes now even come in pre-designed shapes called "precuts." There are special precuts for knees, shoulders, and much more. However, these are primarily intended for use on humans, and are not suitable for animals due to the differences in anatomy—not only are horses' bodies arranged differently from ours, they are also significantly larger. So precuts sized and shaped for human joints are not suitable for taping applications for horses.

Therefore, the classic 5-meter (16.4-foot) tape roll is still the best choice for equine taping. These tapes come in different widths, depending on the manufacturer. The most commonly used is a standard roll 2 inches (5 cm) wide. However, for smaller applications such as scar tapes, there are narrower rolls, and for large areas of musculature, there are correspondingly wider rolls. Again, there is wide variation between manufacturers in terms of the quality of kinesiology tape. Unfortunately, cheap tapes are mostly low quality and do not stick to hair at all, or do stick but only for a very short time. You should definitely seek out a manufacturer who specializes in tape designed for application on animals.

The best way to measure out how much tape you need is to hold the roll up against the horse and see what length of tape you will need for the application you have in mind; then cut the tape to the appropriate shape and size. Almost all manufacturers print lines, or a grid pattern, on the paper backing of the tape, which is a helpful guide for measuring and counting how long each tape strip must be.

Small Pony, Small Tape—Large Horse, Large Tape

You should also consider the differences in size between horses themselves. A Shetland Pony naturally needs smaller, shorter tape strips than a large Holsteiner, and a big draft horse needs much larger pieces of tape than a petite riding pony. Because of these differences in size and the variation in horse breeds, individual measuring tailored to each animal is always necessary. As discussed in chapter 1, kinesiology tape was developed for human use, and the standard tape width of 2 inches has proven to be the most practical for a human-sized body. Fortunately, this is also the ideal width for large animals such as horses and cattle—in most cases. But for very large or very small

Fig. 8.2: The multitude of horse and pony breeds and their wide variation in size require tape strips for each animal and application to be individually measured.

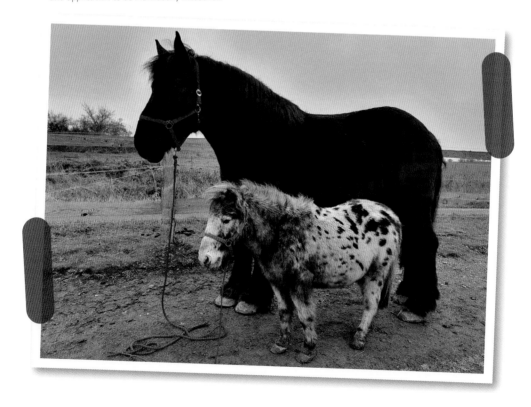

individual animals, it is good to have a few rolls of wider and narrower tape.

Tape Cuts

When using a roll of kinesiology tape, you can cut it into all kinds of shapes and then combine the shapes as you like—and as needed to suit the anatomical structure you are taping.

The most common shapes are the "I" tape, the "Y (or V)" tape and the fan tape. There are some additional tape cuts that are not as common and are only occasionally needed. Of course, the sky is the limit of your own creativity when you are cutting kinesiology tape for your own applications.

The "I" Tape

An "I" tape is a single straight tape strip that is rounded at both ends. It can be used for various applications, and applied with either the end-to-end technique or the inside-out technique. These techniques are described starting on the next page.

The "Y (or V)" Tape

Whether you want to call this tape cut a "Y" or a "V" tape is often down to personal preference, and depends on your individual approach to cutting it, as well as the anatomical structures where it will be used. If your application calls for a smaller closed base, then it will look more like a "V" (as shown in fig. 8.4). If you prefer or find you need to have a larger, longer "trunk," then it will look more like a "Y." That is why this cut has two nicknames.

No matter how you prefer to cut it, this shape of tape always consists of a closed base and two "fingers." Splitting the tape strip into two fingers results in an increase in the surface area you can cover with this tape strip, so you can apply the tape to cover a larger area. The

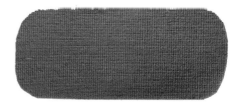

Fig. 8.3: An "I" tape is a single straight tape strip with rounded corners on both ends.

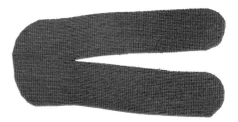

Fig. 8.4: A "Y (or V)" tape always has one closed base and two "fingers," but the length of the base can vary.

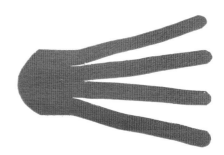

Fig. 8.5: The fan tape always consists of one closed base and multiple tape "fingers."

end-to-end technique is always used for this tape cut.

The Fan Tape

Much like the "Y (or V)" tape, the fan tape also has a single closed base. The special thing about the fan tape cut is that it has several fingers. How many you cut is up to you. Some people always cut three fingers, others four, and others prefer to cut five fingers for a fan tape.

Again, splitting the tape into multiple fingers increases the surface area you can cover. The more fingers you cut, the wider you can spread them, and the larger the area of the body you can cover with them. This tape cut is most often used for hematoma tapes or lymph tapes—when you want to decongest a large swollen area on the abdomen or in the extremities as quickly as possible. It is also used for large fascia problems, or for wider muscles. The end-to-end technique is always used to apply the fan tape.

Taping Techniques

There are essentially only two ways to apply kinesiology tape to a patient. These two techniques are explained here; how they are then used with different tape applications is explained step-by-step in chapters 10 to 20 (starting on page 60).

End-to-End Technique

All fan tapes and all "Y (or V)" tapes are applied with the end-to-end technique. If I Tapes are used for an application such as a muscle taping, for example, they are also applied using the end-to-end technique.

This means that you apply the primary closed base (A) (also called the initial base) first. Then you apply the effective area (B) in the desired direction, and with the amount of stretch needed; the secondary base or final base (C) is applied last.

You work from one end of the tape strip to the other end—hence the name. Since the kinesiology tape will always recoil toward the primary base (A), the contraction in this technique is always pointing in the direction *opposite* the actual application direction of the tape strip.

Example: A muscle taping for the long back muscle is applied from the cranial end, at the withers, to the caudal end, at the highest point of the croup. The primary initial base (A)

Fig. 8.6: Schematic illustration of a tape strip applied with the end-to-end technique. A = the primary base; B = the direction of application; C = the secondary base; arrow = direction of application.

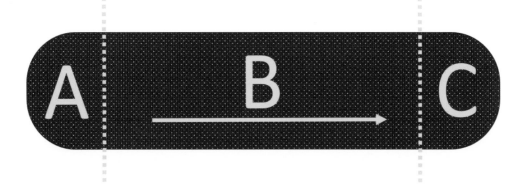

points toward the head (usually at the level of the withers). The effective area (B) then runs along the muscle belly of the long back muscle, parallel to the spine. The secondary end base (C) is located near the sacrum. Applied this way, the kinesiology tape will contract with its recoil directed toward the primary base (A) at the withers.

Inside-Out Technique

This technique is only used for the application of "I" tapes—for example, when applying a decompression tape, a stabilization tape, or a scar tape.

This technique has **NO** primary base. Instead, you hold on to both ends of the tape strip and stretch it from the center out. The effective area (B) is in the center of the tape strip, so in this technique, the tape's recoil is directed toward the center of the tape strip. The ends of the tape strip are both secondary, final bases (C).

Scissors

Next to the kinesiology tape itself, the second most important tool for taping is the scissors! Do not try to save money here. A good pair of scissors is absolutely essential. Since kinesiology tape is made of cotton fabric, cutting it is like trying to cut through a t-shirt or dish towel. You need cutting scissors that are much sharper than regular household scissors. High-quality taping scissors have a titanium coating, too. This coating prevents the adhesive from the kinesiology tape from sticking to the blade when you are cutting the tape. Simple household scissors usually can't cope with cutting tape for very long, and quickly become dull, or else the blades get sticky. So you should always use high-quality taping scissors right from the beginning. Should your specially coated taping scissor blades get sticky from tape adhesive after a lot of use, you can easily clean them with nail polish remover or lighter fluid.

Fig. 8.7: Schematic illustration of a tape strip applied with the inside-out technique. There is no primary base (A)! B = the effective area of the tape strip with the application from the inside out; C = the two secondary bases; arrows = directions of application.

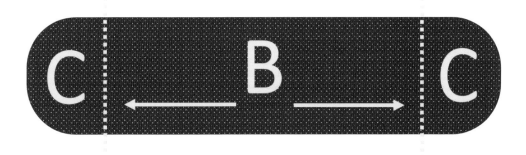

SAFETY NOTE: Taping scissors are really, really sharp! Always take good care of your own fingers when cutting. I have seen some taping students in courses who have cut into their own fingers!

In addition, always turn away from the horse when you are cutting your tape. Even the best horse can get startled and jump off to the side. If your taping scissors are right there, sticking out toward him, it will be a very unpleasant encounter for the horse!

Handling Kinesiology Tape

Rounded Corners

As you could see in all the preceding pictures, the corners of kinesiology tape in a taping application are always rounded, even though the tape comes off the roll with square corners. The corners are deliberately and intentionally cut to make them rounded. This is for the same reason most band-aids have rounded corners: both band-aids and tape are more likely to rub off or fray at the edges if the corners are squared off. Squared corners are practically designed to catch at their tips, whether on your fingers, your clothing, velcro, or a grooming brush. To avoid this, prevent premature detachment, and maximize the amount of time the application stays in place, the corners of the tape strips should be rounded off.

Quick Tip: If you have measured out the required length of tape against the horse, you can fold the length of tape at the center; line up the loose end with the end of the tape that is still attached to the roll, and then trim them both into a rounded shape at the same time, cutting through both layers of tape at once. This saves some time; you've cut your length of tape off the roll and rounded both ends in one go. If you tape a lot, you will quickly come to appreciate this method.

Fig. 8.8: The corners of kinesiology tape strips are rounded to prevent snagging, fraying, and premature detachment. To save a step—and some time—fold the tape over at the center of the required length and shape both ends at the same time!

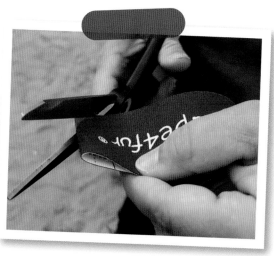

Removing the Paper Backing

Once you have measured and cut an appropriate length of kinesiology tape, the next step is to tear the paper across the back and remove it to expose the adhesive surface. Do *not* try to pick the backing off the tape at the end of the strip! This is tedious and takes longer than it needs to. Instead, tear the paper across the width of the back of the tape with a little twist at the desired spot. Nothing will happen to the tape itself; remember, it's woven fabric, so twisting it won't break it or even weaken it.

If the paper still sticks firmly to the tape at the torn spot and you can't remove it from the tape, then you can simply pull hard on one end of the kinesiology tape—the paper will pop off the tape at the torn spot.

Flat Fingers

Kinesiology tape should always be applied with flat fingers. This results in an even stretch within the tape strip over its complete width. This uses the full recoil potential of the tape, and that allows the greatest possible range of effect to be achieved.

Never stretch or apply the tape with pointed or individual fingers. This will stretch the tape unevenly—it will be stretched much more in the middle, where your thumb or finger is placed on the tape, than at the outer edges above and below that point where you are not holding it. The effects will be equally uneven, and you will not see the results you should.

Stretch-Free Ends

The ends of a tape strip are always applied without any stretch; otherwise, there will be too much tension in the overall application. The more stretch—especially at the ends—the higher the tension within the tape application, and the higher the probability that the

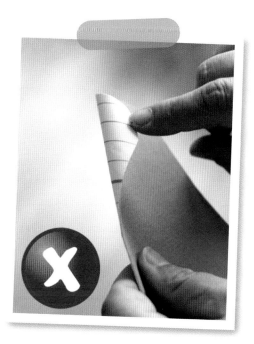

Fig. 8.9: When you are removing the paper backing, don't fumble around trying to peel the paper off at one end of the strip.

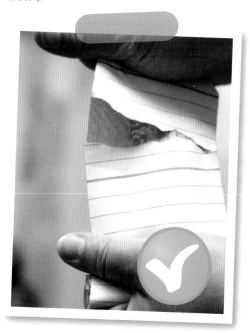

Fig. 8.10: Tear the paper backing completely across with a little twist at the desired spot to remove the paper from the tape.

Preparing and Handling Kinesiology Tape   **47**

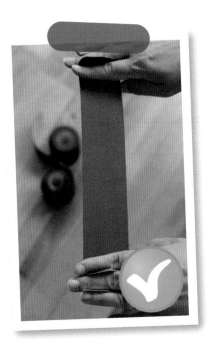

Fig. 8.11: Tape strips are always applied with flat fingers to achieve the best result.

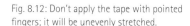

Fig. 8.12: Don't apply the tape with pointed fingers; it will be unevenly stretched.

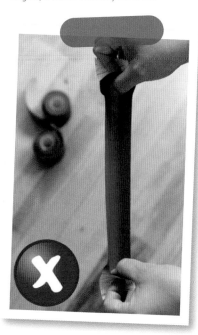

kinesiology tape will start to peel off. It is also helpful if you push these tension-free ends back slightly toward the center of the tape strip once it has been applied. This is known as a "back-up" of the initial or primary and final or secondary bases.

Frictional Heat

Another special feature of the adhesive used for kinesiology tape is that it is activated by heat. Once your taping application is complete, rub vigorously but carefully back and forth over the tape until your own hand gets nice and warm. Rubbing this way creates frictional heat,

which activates the acrylic adhesive of the tape.

Quick Tip: If you live in a location with significant seasonal variation in temperatures, you may not always need to rub your tape the same way. For example, in the northern hemisphere, when it is nice and warm out in the summertime, you don't need to rub over the tape as thoroughly, because the sun will heat it up for you. In the winter, however, vigorous rubbing is very important! During cold weather, if it's an option, you can also position the horse under heated lighting after the tape is applied. The heat will then activate the acrylic adhesive for you.

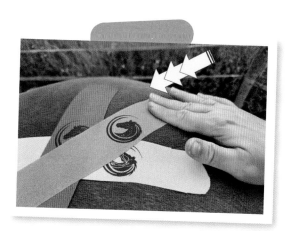

Fig. 8.13: The ends of a tape strip are always applied without any stretch. This effect can be strengthened with a "back-up," indicated by the arrow in the picture.

Non-Reusable

Be aware: Kinesiology tape, once applied, is not reusable in animal therapy. This is especially important to remember if you "mis-tape." If you accidentally do not apply the tape to the affected area correctly on the first try, you can't take it off again, reposition it, and put it back on. There is always a certain amount of dust, skin oil, and loose hair stuck to the adhesive after it has been applied and then peeled off again; once it is contaminated this way, it won't stick well the second time. Even with human patients, it is not really practical to apply the same tape twice—human skin is oily and sheds its cells regularly, both of which affect the adhesive enough that kinesiology tape cannot be reused on us either. So if you are not satisfied with your taping application, the only thing that will fix it is removing the tape again, disposing of it, cutting a new piece, and then applying this new tape in a better position!

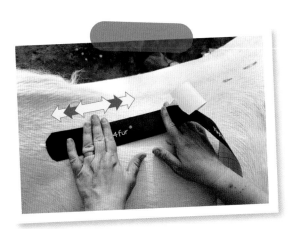

Fig. 8.14: Rubbing over the tape once it is applied creates frictional heat, which fully activates the adhesive capacity of the tape.

Removing the Tape

Kinesiology tape should always be removed from the horse in alignment with the direction of the horse's hair. Some types of tape adhere better than others; in no case should tape be pulled off in a jerky manner. With sensitive horses, this could lead to undesirable reactions—for example, the muscle that was just taped in order to relax it could contract again, due to the pain caused by the rapid, uneven removal of the tape. It is entirely possible for a response like this to completely undo any effect the kinesiology tape might have had. It helps to hold the hair in place with your free hand, or even to press lightly into it, so you do not pull on the hair as you remove the kinesiology tape. Most pain receptors in furred animals are located around the roots of their hair. So if you hold on to the hair a little bit with one hand, you will reduce the degree of tension on the hair roots, and the sensation for the horse will be less unpleasant and less painful.

Occasionally, very fine traces of adhesive may remain on the hair after the kinesiology tape has been removed. These adhesive residues can be easily wiped off with a damp towel and warm water.

How Much Should the Tape Be Stretched?

This is always one of the most common questions. There are taping courses where instructors will talk about 10 percent, 20 percent, 50 percent, or 100 percent stretch in the tape. I think this is unhelpful phrasing. After all, who stands next to the horse stretching their tape with a ruler in hand to measure and calculate the percentage of stretch applied to the tape?

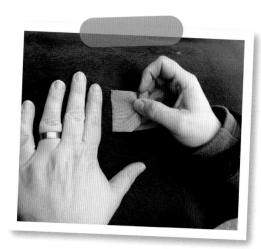

Fig. 8.15: Always remove the tape in alignment with the direction of the hair. With your free hand, hold on to the hair to reduce the tension on the roots.

I prefer the terms "mild," "moderate," and "strong." Naturally, it is a subjective feeling to try to determine which kind of stretch is which, and it takes quite a bit of practice and experience to accurately assess the amount of stretch you have.

I recommend you always keep two things in mind:

1. The softer the tissue, the less stretch you need.
   - Muscles and fascia—mild stretch.
   - Tendons and ligaments—moderate stretch.
   - Bones and joints—strong stretch.
2. The ultimate rule for the stretch in the tape when you are using it on animals: **Less is more!**

Too much stretch in the tape always means too much pull on the hair, the roots of the hair, and the underlying tissue, as well as irritation to the pain receptors in this area. This can cause skin irritation and often feel uncomfortable, and even painful. Human patients can tell their therapist or, if necessary, remove tape from their bodies themselves if it is stretched too much and it feels uncomfortable. Unfortunately, our four-legged patients cannot do this as well as we can. Instead, if the tape is stretched too much, the horse may have a clear defensive reaction to the tape, especially if he is very sensitive. In this case, remove the kinesiology tape immediately, and then reapply the taping with significantly less stretch. It is important to observe the horse after applying a taping. If there is too much tension on the tape, you will often see clear defensive reactions, such as attempts to rub the application off or snapping at the tape with the teeth, almost immediately after the tape is put on.

The classic beginner's mistake is to have too much tension in the tape—since it is so elastic, you are always tempted to stretch it as much as possible. I felt the same way in the beginning, and I see this again and again in my taping courses. It is helpful to try taping yourself before you tape a horse. Cut three pieces of kinesiology tape, all the same length, and apply them next to each other with different degrees of stretch—on your thigh, for example. The first strip should be applied with the 10 percent tension it comes with off the paper backing, the second strip with maximum stretch, and the third tape strip with medium stretch. Usually, within a few minutes, you'll perceive the tape with the most stretch as the most uncomfortable and the one with the least stretch as the most comfortable.

Never forget that the tape is already applied to the paper backing with 10

percent pre-stretch. This 10 percent is often enough for taping horses. The roots of a horse's hair are surrounded by many more sensory cells than we have in our "naked" bare skin, and therefore horses also respond with much more sensitivity to the smallest stimulation!

Even taping applications such as proprioception tapings, which are applied completely without stretch, have an effect, because they influence body perception in the area where they are positioned via the finest shear forces created between tape and the hair! For more specifics, see chapter 20 (page 148).

Anchors

Anchors are mostly simple "I" tapes and are mainly applied across the beginning or end of an application, with absolutely no stretch. They have no impact on the effect of the actual taping application, except insofar as they help it stay on longer: anchors give the taping application better hold, which helps the tape adhere better and gives the application greater longevity. Anchors are also very helpful near joints, if the taping application spans a joint that has a large range of motion.

Important: Anchors are always applied with absolutely no stretch.

How Long Should the Tape Remain on the Horse?

A question I am often asked is, "And how long do the colored strips have to stay on my horse?"

In most cases, I recommend people remove kinesiology tape after about 3–4 days, if the tape does not come off prematurely on its own.

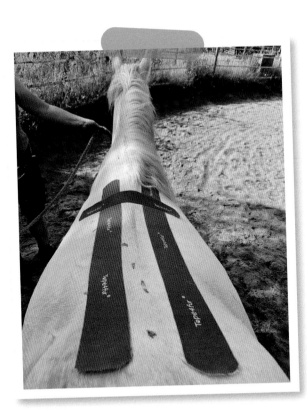

Fig. 8.16: This pink muscle taping for the long back muscle was secured with a blue cross anchor near the withers.

(Reminder: Always peel the tape off in alignment with the grain of the hair.)

Since kinesiology tape in the veterinary field is exposed to wind, weather, hair, and so on, and therefore experiences greater strain than it does when applied to humans, the applications usually do not last long. Some last only a few days, some a week, and now and then there are taping applications that seem to be made for eternity. That's when I get a phone call after 10 to 14 days from the horse owner, asking whether they can take the tape off now! But this is the exception, not the rule.

It is important to keep an eye on the horse to see if he shows any signs of discomfort or is bothered by the tape. In those cases, remove the tape.

The tape has the greatest effect within the first 24 hours. After that, its effectiveness decreases; "habituation" sets in, which is to say the horse, and specifically his receptor cells, get used to the tape. After a few days, the sensation is no longer perceived by the body as "new," and the cells respond less and less strongly to the stimulus of the tape. Most people who have been taped themselves say that after 3 to 4 days, the tape no longer feels "new," and then it can be removed. It is the same with horses.

An exception here is taping applications purely intended to support or augment the effects of training. These are applied for the duration of training only and are removed directly after the session is over.

In Combination with Other Therapeutic Modalities

Kinesiology taping can and should be combined with other therapies, since taping applications are primarily intended as a supportive form of therapy. While massages, lymphatic drainage, acupuncture, stretching exercises, and manual techniques should be used *before* applying the tape, you can also combine taping with a magnetic blanket, TENS, laser, or ultrasound treatment *afterward*. Once applied, as long as it has adhered well, the tape can also get wet, and the horse can be put in a water treadmill, for example, or the legs can be hosed down. But do be careful when drying him off. Carefully dab the taped area dry; do not rub over it vigorously with a towel!

Fig. 8.17: Combining kinesiology tape and a magnetic blanket.

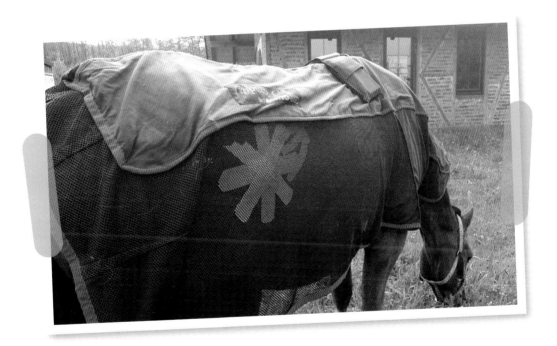

Chapter 9

Before You Begin

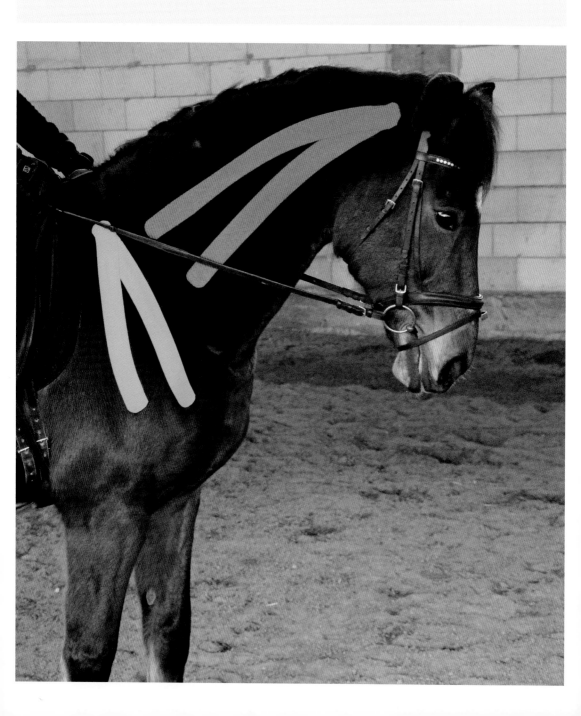

The following chapters describe the taping applications that have proven themselves over the years, the ones that I use most often. Of course, there are more applications than I have included here, and every taping company, school, and method has its own special procedures, not to mention there are no limits to your own creativity. I will only say that you should always check yourself and ask yourself these questions:

- What is the problem my patient is dealing with?

- Can I address the problem with kinesiology taping? If yes, how?

- What do I want to achieve with the taping? What is my goal?

- Which category of structure will I be working on: muscle, fascia, tendons, ligaments, bones, or joints?

- Where exactly is this structure? Where is the beginning and the end? What should I keep in mind about the area around it?

A requirement for a helpful, successful taping application is a detailed, correct diagnosis. Kinesiology taping is a *supportive* treatment modality, and is most effective *in combination* with veterinary care and recommended physiotherapeutic treatments! Kinesiology taping does not replace treatment by a veterinarian or animal physiotherapist.

Again and again, I see pictures of taped horses where I can only wonder what the therapist wanted to achieve. Even after looking at them for a long time, the purposes of some applications still do not become clear to me. Even if treatment through kinesiology taping is still controversial and has not been scientifically proven to be effective, you should not apply kinesiology tape just because it looks pretty. If in doubt, it is better to get the help of an experienced animal physiotherapist with knowledge of taping techniques. They can go over the horse's condition with you and show you exactly which taping applications will achieve the best effect in the case you have brought to them.

I have tried to explain the taping applications in the following chapters in a generally understandable way. However, you cannot do without a few technical terms, so the following pages list the most important anatomy and taping terms at a glance.

Anatomical Terminology

In the descriptions of the taping applications in the following chapters and case studies, I have tried to keep everything clear and easy to understand, and have avoided resorting to technical terminology as much as possible. Still, these words are sometimes unavoidable, especially when it is a choice between more familiar wording or clarity regarding the alignment and direction of the tape on a horse.

Equine Positional and Directional Terms

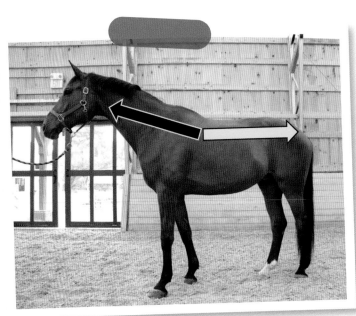

Fig. 9.1:

Blue arrow—the **cranial** direction, which means forward or toward the head.

Yellow arrow—the **caudal** direction, which means backward or toward the tail.

Fig. 9.2:

Blue arrow—the **dorsal** direction, which means toward the upper side, the back, or the topline.

Yellow arrow—the **ventral** direction, which means toward the underside, the belly, or the abdomen.

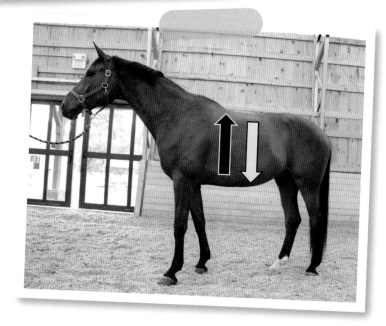

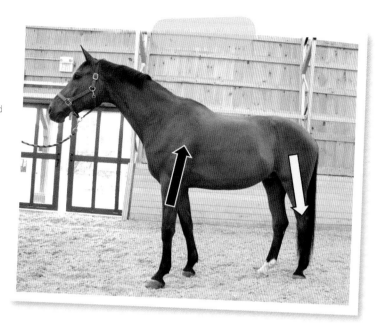

Fig. 9.3:

Blue arrow—the **proximal** direction, which means toward the center of the body.

Yellow arrow—the **distal** direction, which means away from the center of the body.

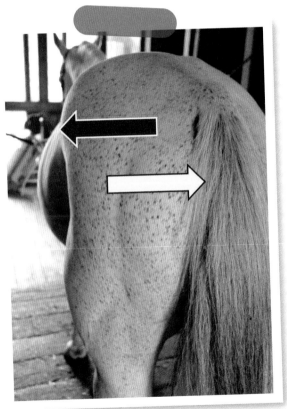

Fig. 9.4:

Blue arrow—the **lateral** direction, which means toward the side or toward the outside.

Yellow arrow—the **medial** direction, which means toward the center or toward the middle.

Anatomical Terms for Muscles

Hypertonic: Higher or elevated muscle tone or tension.

Hypotonic: Reduced or lowered muscle tone or tension.

Hypertrophic: Overdeveloped, enlarged muscle.

Atrophic: Underdeveloped, reduced muscle.

Myogelosis or **trigger point:** An area or point with palpable and painful chronic tense musculature.

Spasm: A sudden, involuntary, painful muscle contraction.

Taping Terminology

There are also a few technical terms relating to the kinesiology tape rather than the horse that will be used again and again, and which I would therefore like to discuss in more detail.

Back-Up

The back-up could also be described as a "push back." A back-up in horse taping always takes place when the stretch-free ends of the taping strips are applied to the hair. It does not matter whether the stretch-free end is at the beginning or the end of the taping strip.

If you apply a strip of kinesiology tape in the direction of the grain of the horse's coat with the end-to-end technique, you are applying the beginning of the tape strip without any stretch, and at the same time you push this piece of tape back slightly, against the direction of the coat, with the palm of your hand or your fingers, held flat—that motion against the direction of the coat is the back-up. This reinforces the effect of the stretch- and tension-free beginning of the application. The same procedure is used at the end of the tape strip. The middle section of the tape strip is applied with the desired stretch up to approximately the last 2 inches. Any pre-stretch is released from this secondary end, and it is also pushed back slightly against the direction of the coat—a second back-up.

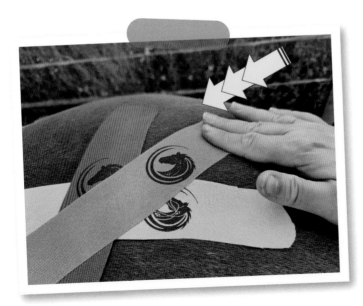

Fig. 9.5: When applying the "back-up," you are pushing each end of the tape strip slightly backward (toward the center of the tape strip) to make sure the end is absolutely stretch-free.

If kinesiology tape is applied with the inside-out technique, both ends of each tape strip are also applied without any stretch or tension. The back-up, however, takes place in the direction of the center of the tape strip (so the ends of the strip move toward each other during the back-up, rather than in the same direction as described above).

Recoil

As you now know, kinesiology tape is elastic and stretchable, and is applied to the patient with a specific amount of stretch. Everything that is stretched has a tendency to try to contract back to its original unstretched shape. This effort to contract is called "recoil" in kinesiology taping. Keep this recoil effect in mind with each taping application—figuring out what you want to achieve with the tape includes thinking about which direction you want the recoil to be angled, and therefore which direction you want the tape angled, too.

With the end-to-end technique, recoil is always directed toward the primary base of the tape strip. This means the direction of recoil is always opposite the direction in which you applied the tape. With the inside-out technique, recoil is always directed toward the center of the tape strip.

As an example, consider a muscle taping to support muscle contraction. In this case, the recoil must be aimed in the same direction in which the targeted muscle contracts. If you

wanted to support relaxation and stretching of the muscle instead, then you would want to aim the recoil in the same direction in which that muscle stretches.

Another example to think about is a lymph taping. To encourage drainage of trapped fluid, the recoil must be aimed away from the swelling and toward the lymph node.

The direction of the tape and its recoil will be covered in more detail in each of the following chapters describing application techniques, but this should give you some idea of the basic principles involved.

One More Important Note before We Get Going!

The advice, taping applications, and other recommendations in this book were written to the best of my knowledge and carefully checked. However, no guarantees can be given. Neither I as the author nor the publishers of this book can be held liable for personal injury, property damage, or financial loss.

In addition, I would like to point out that all medical and therapeutic treatments are constantly changing, thanks to modern research, new findings, and the results of scientific exploration. This applies to kinesiology taping, too. The techniques and effects described in this book correspond to the current state of knowledge regarding kinesiology taping for horses.

Chapter 10

Muscle Taping

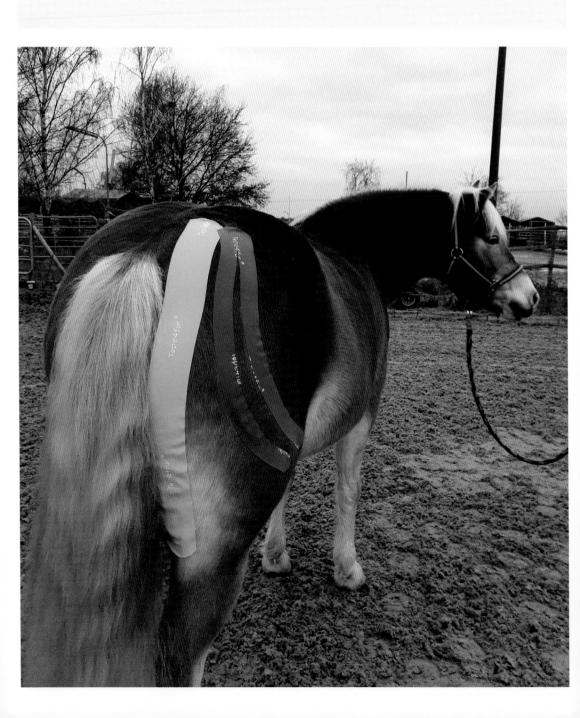

Muscles

There are three types of muscles in the bodies of almost every mammal.

- **Smooth muscles:** These are controlled by the autonomic nervous system and cannot be controlled or directed voluntarily. This includes, for example, the muscles in the intestinal system.

- **Cardiac muscles:** These are controlled independently by the cardiac sinus node, and are really only found in the heart. Much like smooth muscles, these cannot be controlled at will.

- **Skeletal muscles:** These are what most people picture when you say the word "muscle"—the muscles attached to the skeleton by tendons, spanning one or sometimes two joints. When these muscles contract, the muscle *belly* shortens, causing the bones where the muscle's ends are attached to move closer together, and making the joint spanned by the muscle *flex*. We can voluntarily contract and relax our skeletal muscles ourselves. These muscles are responsible for movement and locomotion.

The skeletal muscles are the ones we can and want to influence with kinesiology tape. Each of these muscles consists of a tendon of origin, a muscle belly, and a tendon of insertion. The tendons serve to attach the muscle to bones, and the muscle belly performs the contraction. Together, tendons and a muscle always span at least one articulated joint.

A muscle belly consists of many muscle *fibers*, which are themselves composed of thousands of even smaller *myofibrils*. When the muscle is flexed, these fibrils glide past each other, and the muscle shortens, bringing the bones the muscle attaches to closer together; that is how movement occurs. Obviously this explanation is simplifying the process considerably, and it is actually much more complicated. But this covers the basic principles that govern muscle activity.

For any muscle taping application, it is important for you to know where the origin and insertion of the muscle you are targeting are positioned. The origin point is usually proximal—closer to the body—and attached to the less mobile bone. The insertion is typically

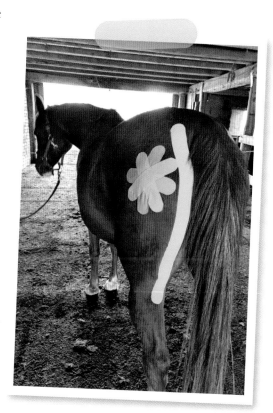

Fig. 10.1: The hamstrings (*M. semitendinosus* and *M. semimembranosus*) are located along the back of the thigh and the femur bone. They are covered with one long apple-green tape strip in this picture.

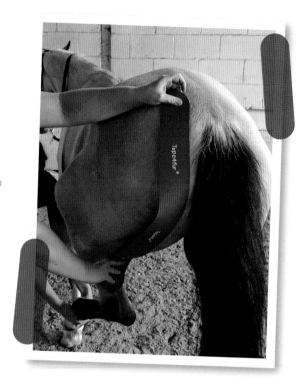

Fig. 10.2: Measuring the appropriate length for a tape strip while pre-stretching the muscle.

distal—farther from the center of the body—and attached to the more mobile bone.

As an example, let's take the semitendinosus muscle, also known as the hamstrings, which is a strong, fleshy muscle that forms the back contour of the thigh. In the horse, this muscle originates at the last sacral vertebra, as well as the first and second tail vertebrae, and also ventrally at the tuber ischia (the point of the buttock). Then comes the muscle belly, which spans both the hip joint and the stifle joint caudally, and can usually also be seen and palpated there very well. The tendinous attachment of the insertion is divided into two parts: one is positioned on the tibia, which allows flexion of the stifle in the swing phase of the leg, and the other runs out into the calcaneal tendon, allowing extension of the hip, stifle, and hock joints in the stance phase of the leg.

Muscle taping can be used to enhance the effects of massage and stretching exercises to relax the muscles, or during training to increase activation of the muscles.

How to Apply a Muscle Taping

For a muscle taping application, *always* use the **end-to-end technique**—you will always be taping either from the origin to the insertion of the muscle, or from the insertion to the origin.

In general, you should pre-stretch the muscle you want to work on. Continuing our previous example of the hamstrings, you will need an assistant to lift the leg, flex it, and bring it as far forward under the belly as the horse will allow.

Other examples: Before taping the long back muscle, it is helpful to bring the horse's nose to the ground, and when taping the neck muscles, you should ask the horse to stretch his neck toward the side opposite the area you will be taping.

I recommend that you always have a helper or the horse's owner present during muscle taping, so there is someone around who can help guide the horse into a bend or hold his leg up if necessary.

- In the aforementioned pre-stretched position for the hamstrings, measure the length of kinesiology tape you will need. Set the leg back down, and give the helper a little break: take a moment to cut the measured tape into an "I" strip with rounded corners.

- Then have the leg picked up again, into the same position as before, and keep the leg or muscle in this pre-stretched position during the application.

- Tear the paper completely across the back of the tape, and remove 1–2 inches of the paper from one end of the "I" tape. Apply this end (called the primary base) first, without any stretch at all, at the origin of the muscle, and then push it back slightly in the direction of the insertion—the back-up.

- Then remove the paper backing completely, except for the last 2 inches at the other end of the "I". Make sure the adhesive side, which is now exposed, does not come into contact with the horse's hair yet.

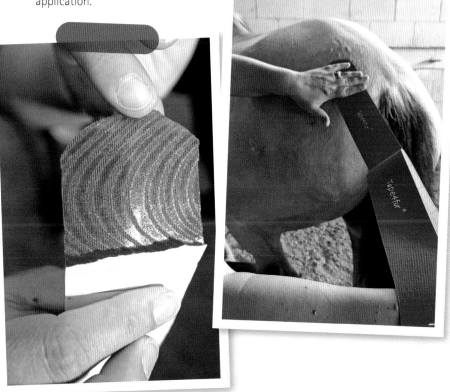

Figs. 10.3 and 10.4: The primary base should be about 2 inches long, and will always be applied without any stretch.

- Hold the tape with flat, straight fingers, and then, with a mild stretch (about 10 percent, the same amount of stretch it had with the paper on), align it along the muscle in the direction of the muscle insertion, and apply it with the other hand, also held flat.

- Then remove the backing from those last 2 inches of tape, and apply this end—again, completely without any stretch, and with a back-up, pushing it back toward the muscle belly.

- Rub vigorously but carefully back and forth over the tape strip (be especially careful at the ends!) to activate the adhesive. After that, the leg can be set down again, and the muscle can be returned to its normal position.

When the muscle is returned to its original position after the tape has been applied—in this case, when the leg is placed back on the ground—waves usually appear within the tape. Do not get nervous! This is how it is supposed to be. These are called "convolutions," and they increase the pull of the taping application and cause an even better "lifting effect." In order to avoid removing these convolutions, I strongly recommend rubbing over the tape when the muscle is still in its pre-stretched position, not waiting until the area has returned to its normal position or the leg is on the ground again and then rubbing—if you rub after these convolutions form, you will compress them and they will no longer augment the lifting effect of the tape.

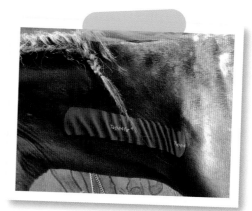

Fig. 10.6: "Convolutions" help enhance the lifting effect of kinesiology tape.

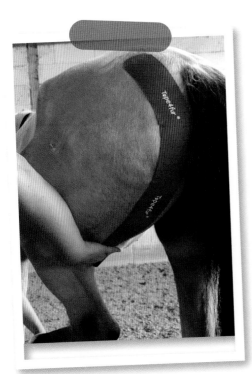

Fig. 10.5: Applying the tape strip while pre-stretching the muscle.

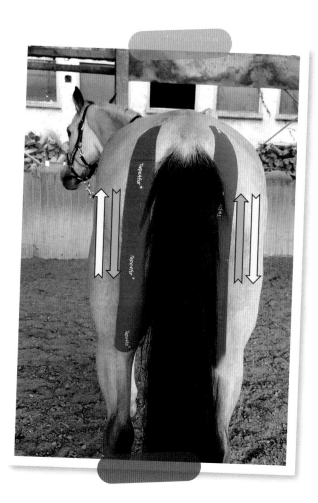

Fig. 10.7: Direction of application and recoil for activation (red tape) and relaxation (blue tape) of the hamstrings.

Activation or Relaxation of Muscles

In light of the structure of skeletal muscle as described above, with its origin and insertion and its ability to contract, there are two possible purposes for taping applications: activation and support of muscle contraction, or relaxation and stretching of muscle. Both of these goals can be achieved with the end-to-end technique.

When a muscle is contracting, as the muscle fibers inside it shorten, the more mobile of the bones it is attached to—usually the bone farther from the body—moves with it, closer to the less mobile bone. In our hamstring example,

when the hamstrings contract, the more mobile thigh bone is brought closer to the less mobile pelvis: the leg is bent.

As a muscle stretches and relaxes, and its fibers lengthen again, its origin and insertion move away from each other, and the more mobile bone moves away from the less mobile bone; in our hamstring example, the leg straightens out into an extended position again.

To **activate** a muscle (red tape), you tape with a mild stretch from the origin to the insertion of the muscle (the green arrow indicates the direction in which to apply the tape). Because of the stretch, the tape will try to contract in the direction of the starting point, which in this case is the muscle origin. This is the same as the direction in which the muscle contracts, so the recoil is supporting contraction of the muscle (the yellow arrow indicates both the direction in which the muscle contracts and the direction of the tape's recoil).

To **relax** a muscle (blue tape), you tape with a mild stretch from the insertion to the origin of the muscle (the green arrow indicates the direction in which to apply the tape). The tape will then try to contract in the direction of the muscle insertion—the opposite direction from that in which the muscle contracts—and this

recoil force therefore supports stretching and relaxation of the muscle (the yellow arrow indicates both the direction in which the muscle stretches and the direction of the tape's recoil).

Based on my own experience, I use the same approach as for muscle activation on mildly to moderately tight muscles; in these cases, I still want to support muscle contraction and improve muscle activity, so it is helpful to give the muscle an impulse for contraction with the tape.

However, if a muscle is highly tense and hard, I use a relaxation taping application.

Muscle taping for activation of the hamstrings:
Direction of application: From origin to insertion.
Recoil: From insertion to origin.
Effect: Activation and contraction of the hamstrings.

Muscle taping for relaxation of the hamstrings:
Direction of application: From insertion to origin.
Recoil: From origin to insertion.
Effect: Relaxation and stretching of the hamstrings.

Unilateral versus Bilateral Muscle Taping

I am a great advocate of *bilateral* muscle taping. Bilateral taping means that even if the problem is only on one side—for example, the horse has a tense back muscle on the left—I will tape both the left back muscle and the right back muscle. In my experience, horses have a tendency to become uneven otherwise, and with riding and sport horses in daily training in particular, this is undesirable. For horses on stall rest, which get little exercise and are therefore stiffer, if they have only one tense area, I occasionally make an exception and tape only on that side. However, in these cases, problems usually occur on both sides anyway.

Be aware: If you have taped the horse's muscles on both sides and the tape comes off on one side but not the other, you should remove the tape on the other side yourself to avoid irregularities and unevenness!

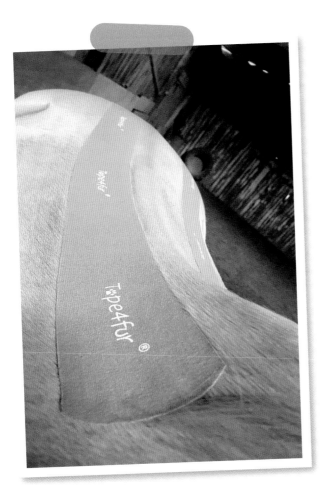

Fig. 10.8: Bilateral muscle taping for the long back muscle.

More Examples of Muscle Taping

All of the following case studies and taping applications are *supportive* measures intended to complement veterinary, physiotherapeutic, or osteopathic treatments!

Gluteal Muscle (*M. gluteus*)

The superficial gluteal muscle originates from the lumbar and gluteal fascia at the level of the lumbar vertebrae, and has its insertion laterally at the upper part of the femur. It flexes the hip joint and moves the hind leg forward. Pre-stretching of this muscle is not necessary because its range of motion is much smaller than that of our example muscle, the hamstrings.

Since the gluteal muscle belly is quite broad, it is difficult to cover it with only one tape strip. The most effective way to deal with this fact is to apply one tape strip along the upper edge of the muscle belly (the yellow tape strip in the photo) and a second strip along the lower edge (the blue tape strip in the photo). You can do this either with two separate "I" tapes or with a "V (or Y)" tape. For very large horses such as draft horses, you can also apply a third strip along the middle of the muscle.

The primary and secondary bases are applied with no stretch; the effective area is applied with mild stretch.

> **Activation and support for contraction of the gluteal muscle:**
> **Direction of application:** From the lumbar and gluteal fascia toward the femur.
> **Recoil:** From the femur toward the lumbar and gluteal fascia.

> **Relaxation and support for stretching of the gluteal muscle:**
> **Direction of application:** From the femur to the lumbar and gluteal fascia.
> **Recoil:** From the lumbar and gluteal fascia to the femur.

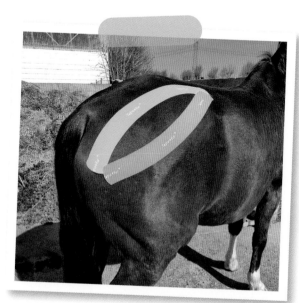

Fig. 10.9: A taping application for the gluteal muscles, using two "I" tapes.

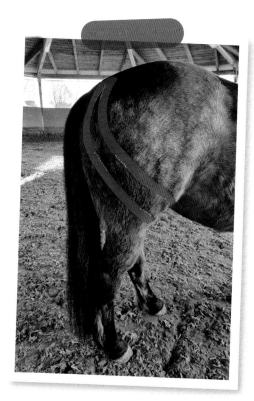

Fig. 10.10: A taping application to activate the thigh muscle, using a "V (or Y)" tape.

Thigh (*M. biceps femoris*)

This thigh muscle has its origin at the last three spinous and transverse processes of the sacrum, as well as at the tuber ischia, and its insertion is at the patella, as well as at the cranial edge of the tibia and laterally at the calcaneal tuberosity. In the stance phase of a horse's movement, it extends the hip, stifle, and hock joints. In the swing phase, it extends the hip and hock joints and flexes the stifle.

To pre-stretch this muscle, have the leg brought forward under the horse's abdomen by a helper. Since the muscle runs out quite broadly toward the stifle, you can work with two to three "I" tapes, or with a "V (or Y)" tape or a fan tape. Which cuts will work the best also depends a bit on the size of the horse and the strength of his hindquarters.

The primary and secondary bases are applied with no stretch; the effective area is applied with mild stretch.

Activation and support for contraction of the thigh muscle:
Direction of application: From the caudal edge of the sacrum to the stifle and stifle fascia.
Recoil: From the stifle toward the caudal edge of the sacrum.

Relaxation and support for stretching of the thigh muscle:
Direction of application: From the stifle toward the caudal edge of the sacrum.
Recoil: From the caudal edge of the sacrum to the stifle and stifle fascia.

TFL (*M. tensor fasciae latae*)

This muscle originates at the point of the hip, and its insertion fuses with the femoral fascia at the level of the stifle and thigh. It flexes the hip joint, and assists in moving the hind leg forward. For taping applications, the leg should be stretched backward by a helper to pre-stretch the muscle. Again, we are dealing with a rather broad muscle, and you can use multiple "I" tapes, multiple "V (or Y)" tapes, or a fan tape.

The primary and secondary bases are applied with no stretch; the effective area is applied with mild stretch.

Activation and support for contraction of the TFL:
Direction of application: From the point of the hip toward the femoral fascia and the stifle.
Recoil: From the stifle to the point of the hip.

Relaxation and support for stretching of the TFL:
Direction of application: From the stifle to the point of the hip.
Recoil: From the point of the hip toward the femoral fascia and the stifle.

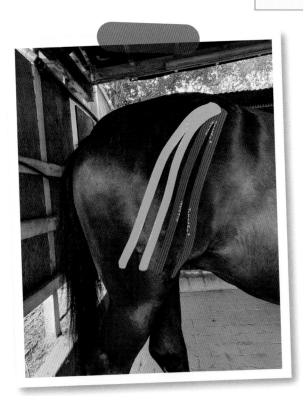

Fig. 10.11: Activation of the TFL, using two "V (or Y)" tapes.

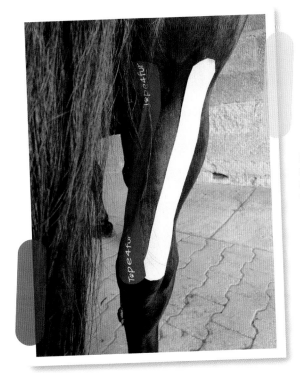

Fig. 10.12: A calf muscle taping application that runs from the cap of the hock to the back of the stifle, to support stretch and elongation.

Calf (*M. gastrocnemius*)

The calf muscle originates medially and laterally at the back of the femur, and has its insertion through the Achilles tendon at the cap of the hock. It flexes the stifle and extends the hock at the same time. This muscle is pre-stretched by flexing the hock as far as possible and moving the leg slightly forward under the horse's abdomen. You can use either two "I" tapes or one "V (or Y)" tape.

The primary and secondary bases are applied with no stretch; the effective area is applied with mild stretch.

Activation and support for contraction of the calf muscle:
Direction of application: From the back of the stifle to the cap of the hock.
Recoil: From the cap of the hock toward the back of the stifle.

Relaxation and support for stretching of the calf muscle:
Direction of application: From the cap of the hock toward the back of the stifle.
Recoil: From the back of the stifle to the cap of the hock.

Straight Abdominal (*M. rectus abdominis*)
The straight abdominal muscle originates on the right and left sides of the fourth through ninth ribs, and has its insertion on the pelvic bone at the level of the pubic symphysis. An application that runs all the way to the pubic symphysis is difficult to tape, because horses are often very sensitive in that area, they do not have much hair there for the tape to stick to, and you would have to crawl under the horse's belly to reach it, too. I usually only go as far as the area where the hair ends, just past the navel.

This muscle has multiple functions, including bearing the weight of the horse's intestines, but in terms of movement, its contraction curves the spine and arches it upward (the same way contraction of muscles in the human abdomen during a sit-up curves our backs toward our knees). It is the counterpart of the long back muscle. It is difficult to pre-stretch this muscle; fortunately, pre-stretching is also not necessary, because this muscle's range of motion is not very big. I recommend you apply a wide "I" tape or a "V (or Y)" tape lengthwise on both the right and left sides of the abdominal midline.

The primary and secondary bases are applied with no stretch; the effective area is applied with mild stretch.

Activation and support for contraction of the straight abdominal muscle:
Direction of application: From the girth area to the caudal edge of the hair.
Recoil: From the edge of the hair toward the girth area.

Relaxation and support for stretching of the straight abdominal muscle:
Direction of application: From the edge of the hair toward the girth area.
Recoil: From the girth area to the caudal edge of the hair.

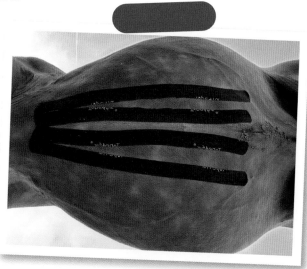

Fig. 10.13: Muscle taping to activate the straight abdominal muscle on both sides, using "V (or Y)" tapes.

Oblique Abdominal (*M. obliquus externus abdominis*)

This very broad muscle originates laterally at the ribs, starting from the fourth or fifth rib, and then extends into the abdominal fascia, which attaches to the abdominal midline. It too carries the weight of the intestines; it also facilitates breathing through its connection to the ribs. To pre-stretch this muscle, a helper can flex the horse to opposite sides—for example, through lateral carrot-stretch exercises. But this muscle's range of motion is also fairly small, and I sometimes tape it without pre-stretching. Since this muscle is very wide, multiple "I" tapes are used.

The primary and secondary bases are applied with no stretch; the effective area is applied with mild stretch.

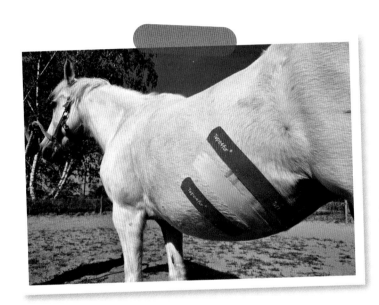

Fig. 10.14: A taping application for the oblique abdominal muscle.

Activation and support for contraction of the oblique abdominal muscle:
Direction of application: From the caudal end of the ribs toward the abdominal midline.
Recoil: From the abdominal midline toward the caudal end of the ribs.

Relaxation and support for stretching of the oblique abdominal muscle:
Direction of application: From the abdominal midline toward the caudal end of the ribs.
Recoil: From the caudal end of the ribs toward the abdominal midline.

Long Back Muscle (*M. longissimus dorsi*)

This muscle has its origin at the cranial edge on the right and left sides of the pelvis, as well as at the spinous processes of the sacrum and the lumbar and caudal thoracic vertebrae. The insertions are found at the transverse processes of the vertebrae, as well as the tops of the ribs. The muscle itself reaches all the way to the occipital bone. However, at the level of the withers, the shoulder blades are positioned above the muscle, and in the neck area, it is covered by other muscles. Therefore, we can really only reach this muscle with kinesiology tape along the length of the back.

The long back muscle is used to brace and stretch the back, and when the hindquarters are planted on the ground, it is responsible for straightening the upper body (for example, when the horse is rearing). This muscle is best pre-stretched by having the horse come down to the ground with his nose, and you can let him stay there and eat a bit of hay from the ground while you are applying the tape. Due to the width of this muscle, I recommend you use tape wider than the standard 2 inches for most horses. Since this muscle lies in a relatively straight line, "I" tapes are used.

The primary and secondary bases are applied with no stretch; the effective area is applied with mild stretch.

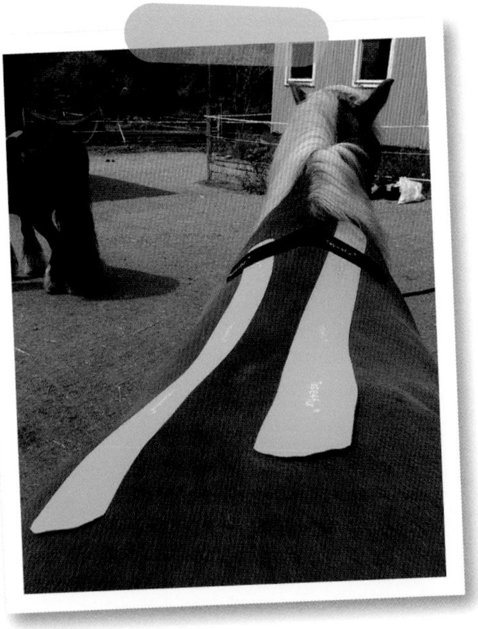

Fig. 10.15: Taping application for relaxation on the long back muscle from the withers toward the pelvis.

Activation and support for contraction of the long back muscle:
Direction of application: From the highest point of the croup to the caudal edge of the shoulder blade.
Recoil: From the shoulder blade to the pelvis.

Relaxation and support for stretching of the long back muscle:
Direction of application: From the caudal edge of the withers to the highest point of the croup.
Recoil: From the pelvis to the withers.

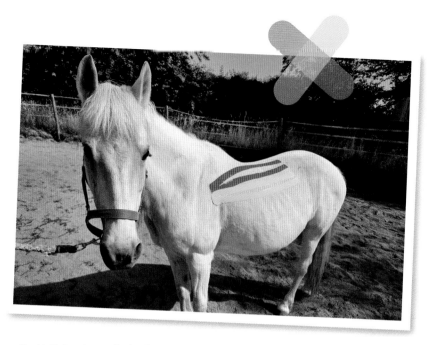

Fig. 10.16: A taping application for the broad back muscle to support stretching and relaxation.

Broad Back Muscle (*M. latissimus dorsi*)

The broad back muscle, as the name suggests, is wide; its origin is in the thoraco-lumbar back fascia, and its insertion is at the humerus. When the horse is in motion, it is responsible for pulling the forelimb backward and flexing the shoulder joint. When the forehand is planted, flexing it pulls the trunk forward. The best way to pre-stretch this muscle is to have a helper hold up the foreleg and draw it forward into a stretch. Since its origin is very wide, I recommend either several "I" tapes, several "V (or Y)" tapes, or a large fan tape.

The primary and secondary bases are applied with no stretch; the effective area is applied with mild stretch.

Activation and support for contraction of the broad back muscle:
Direction of application: From the lumbar fascia toward the humerus.
Recoil: From the humerus to the lumbar fascia.

Relaxation and support for stretching of the broad back muscle:
Direction of application: From the humerus to the lumbar fascia.
Recoil: From the lumbar fascia toward the humerus.

Trapezius (*M. trapezius*)

The trapezius muscle has a very wide origin along the nuchal ligament of the neck and the thoracic spine, and has its insertion along the scapular spine on the shoulder blade. It raises the forelimb, and assists in leading the leg forward or sideways (in lateral gaits). To tape the caudal section of the muscle in the thoracic spine, pre-stretch it by moving the horse's head diagonally downward to the opposite side. For the cranial section in the neck, pre-stretch it by guiding the horse's head to the opposite side. The cervical and thoracic portions of this muscle can be taped separately, or at the same time.

This muscle, as noted, is very wide, and therefore several individual "I" tapes or fan tapes are recommended here as well.

The primary and secondary bases are applied with no stretch; the effective area is applied with mild stretch.

Activation and support for contraction of the trapezius muscle:
Direction of application: From the nuchal ligament to the scapular spine on the shoulder blade.
Recoil: From the scapular spine on the shoulder blade to the nuchal ligament.

Relaxation and support for stretching of the trapezius muscle:
Direction of application: From the scapular spine on the shoulder blade to the nuchal ligament.
Recoil: From the nuchal ligament toward the shoulder blade.

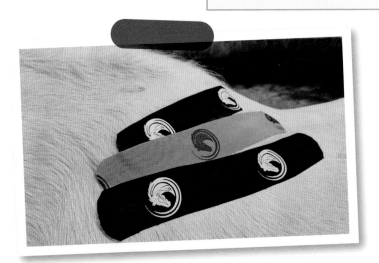

Fig. 10.17: A taping application to activate the caudal part of the trapezius muscle in the area of the thoracic spine and withers.

Triceps (*M. triceps brachii*)

The triceps originates at the caudal edge of the scapula, as well as medially and laterally on the humerus, and attaches to the olecranon at the point of the main foreleg joint (the horse's "elbow," so to speak). Primarily, it extends the elbow joint and assists in flexing the shoulder joint. This muscle can be pre-stretched by bringing the target leg forward into the greatest possible flexion, with the carpal joint flexed as well. Since the origin of the triceps is quite wide, I recommend you tape this muscle with several "I" tapes or a fan tape.

The primary and secondary bases are applied with no stretch; the effective area is applied with mild stretch.

Activation and support for contraction of the thigh muscle:
Direction of application: From the caudal edge of the shoulder blade toward the elbow.
Recoil: From the elbow to the shoulder blade.

Relaxation and support for stretching of the thigh muscle:
Direction of application: From the elbow toward the caudal edge of the shoulder blade.
Recoil: From the shoulder blade toward the elbow.

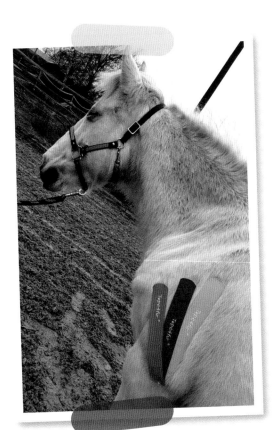

Fig. 10.18: A relaxing muscle taping application for the triceps, from the point of the horse's "elbow" to the caudal edge of the shoulder blade.

Infraspinatus and Supraspinatus (*M. supraspinatus* and *M. infrasprinatus*)

These two muscles are so close together and function so similarly that I will describe them together in this section. They can be taped together, or only one of the two can be taped if only one is affected by a specific issue.

They originate at the scapular cartilage, which is positioned at the dorsal edge of the scapula at the withers. The supraspinatus then runs through the cranial scapulothoracic fossa, in front of the scapular spine; the infraspinatus runs through the caudal scapulothoracic fossa, behind the scapular spine. Both have their insertion at the head of the humerus. They assist in extension of the shoulder joint, but mainly they serve to stabilize it. Pre-stretching of these muscles is not really necessary because their range of motion is so small.

Since they are both fairly straight, it is best to use one "I" tape per muscle, or one "V (or Y)" tape that covers both muscles at once.

The primary and secondary bases are applied with no stretch; the effective area is applied with mild stretch.

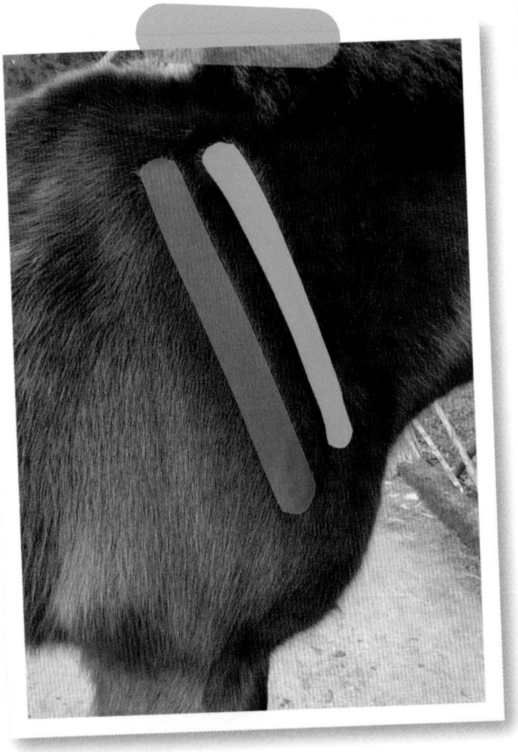

Fig. 10.19: An activation taping for the supraspinatus and infraspinatus muscles, running from the scapular cartilage at the withers to the shoulder joint.

Activation and support for contraction of the supraspinatus and infraspinatus:
Direction of application: From the scapular cartilage at the withers toward the shoulder joint.
Recoil: From the shoulder to the withers.

Relaxation and support for stretching of the supraspinatus and infraspinatus:
Direction of application: From the shoulder joint toward the scapular cartilage at the withers.
Recoil: From the withers toward the shoulder.

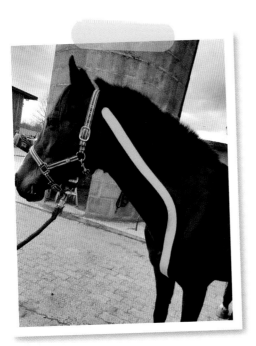

Fig. 10.20: A taping application for the brachiocephalic muscle, running from the wing of the atlas toward the shoulder joint, to assist with forward movement of the front limb.

Activation and support for lifting and forward movement of the front limb:
Direction of application: From the wing of the atlas toward the shoulder joint.
Recoil: From the shoulder toward the back of the head.

Activation and support for lowering and lateral flexion of the head and neck:
Direction of application: From the shoulder joint toward the wing of the atlas.
Recoil: From the back of the head toward the shoulder.

Brachiocephalic Muscle
(*M. brachiocephalicus*)

The brachiocephalic muscle is a very complex muscle; it runs between the end of the humerus (in the area of the shoulder) and the back of the head. Anatomically, it is subdivided again, depending on where it originates and attaches. The most important portion of this muscle in the context of kinesiology taping originates at the clavicular strip directly above the shoulder joint, and has its attachment at the occipital bone.

This muscle has two functions and can work in either direction! In the stance phase of the horse's movement, it pulls his head down and to the side, when contracted unilaterally. In the swing phase, it lifts his forelimb and leads it upward and forward. Therefore, when you are taping this muscle, it is always important to consider which movement you want to support, and thus in which direction you want to tape (see the descriptions in blue text below). With this muscle, it is very important to pre-stretch it to the opposite side no matter what you want to achieve with your taping application, as the range of motion of this muscle is very large. Since the brachiocephalic muscle is very straight, it is best to use wide "I" tapes for this.

The primary and secondary bases are applied with no stretch; the effective area is applied with mild stretch.

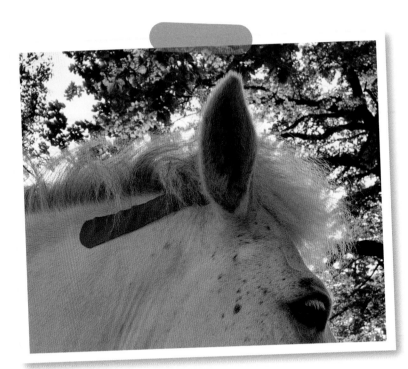

Fig. 10.21: A muscle taping to relax the straight neck muscle, running from the back of the neck toward the second vertebra.

Straight Neck Muscle (*M. rectus capitis*)
The straight neck muscle originates dorsally at the second cervical vertebra and has its insertion at the occipital bone. It raises the horse's head and stretches his upper neck. Pre-stretching this muscle can be a bit tricky, as there is often a lot of tension here, and the horse has to come down with his nose as far as he can toward the sternum, flexing his neck as much as possible. "I" tapes are used for this muscle.

The primary and secondary bases are applied with no stretch; the effective area is applied with mild stretch.

Activation and support for contraction of the straight neck muscle:
Direction of application: From the second vertebra to the occipital bone.
Recoil: From the back of the head toward the second vertebra.

Relaxation and support for stretching of the straight neck muscle:
Direction of application: From the occipital bone to the second vertebra.
Recoil: From the second vertebra toward the back of the head.

Masseter (*M. masseter*)

The masseter muscle originates at the cheek-bone in the upper jaw, spans the upper and lower molars, and has its insertion at the ventral edge of the lower jaw. It is responsible for muscular action during chewing; it lifts the lower jaw and presses it against the upper jaw. Pre-stretching it is somewhat difficult, as the horse would have to open his mouth and keep it open to stretch this area. However, since the masseter's range of motion is rather small, pre-stretching is not really necessary. The masseter muscle is quite wide, so use either parallel "I" tapes or a fan tape.

The primary and secondary bases are applied with no stretch; the effective area is applied with mild stretch.

Activation and support for contraction of the masseter muscle:
Direction of application: From the cheekbone toward the ventral edge of the lower jaw.
Recoil: From the lower jaw toward the cheekbone.

Relaxation and support for stretching of the masseter muscle:
Direction of application: From the ventral edge of the lower jaw toward the cheekbone.
Recoil: From the cheekbone toward the lower jaw.

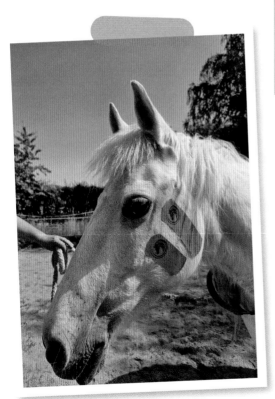

Fig. 10.22: An activating muscle tape for the masseter, with two parallel "I" tapes running from the cheek bone to the ventral edge of the lower jaw.

Chapter 11

Fascia Taping

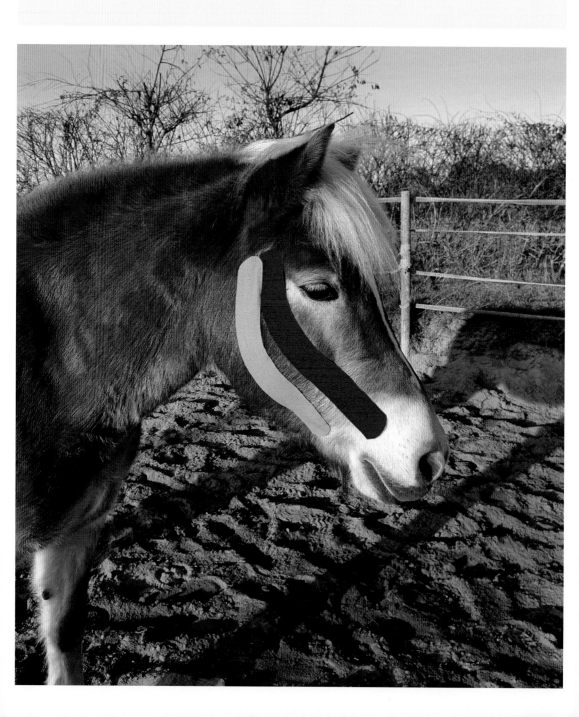

The Fascia

Fasciae are a kind of connective tissue. In contrast to scar tissue, which will be discussed in Chapter 17, fasciae are not firm or inelastic. On the contrary: fasciae are flexible parallel layers of connective tissue, which surround muscles, muscle fibers, and organs. Most areas of fascia are thin, but there are also very thick fascia—for example, the thoracic-lumbar fascia in the horse's back.

Fasciae serve as a protective layer. The fascia around the muscles also ensure that muscles and muscle fibers can glide smoothly

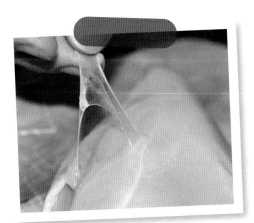

Fig. 11.1: The wafer-thin fascia layer of a chicken breast that is ready to be cooked.

past each other during both contraction and stretching.

In the past, little attention was paid to fasciae, and they were considered uninteresting connective tissues. In recent years, however, much research has been done on them, and we have learned that these extremely thin structures are enormously important to the body. They are permeated with sensory and nerve cells, and play a major role in proprioception. Many researchers now call fascia an independent organ, and some even go as far as to consider it the most important organ of the body.

For all readers who have ever cut up a chicken breast while cooking, you may have noticed the meat is usually surrounded by a whitish, translucent layer of tissue. This is the fascia.

As noted, fasciae usually glide smoothly, but they can become stuck together due to trauma or permanent or extreme stress, and then they can no longer move as they should, which will eventually have a negative effect on muscle activity, and on the whole organism.

These "stuck" fasciae can be loosened by special techniques and massages—and fascia taping applications are a great option as support for manual fascia-related techniques.

How to Apply a Fascia Taping

This form of taping aims to reorganize stuck, tight, or restricted fascia and help restore it to its original functional state. There are two ways to approach taping applications for this purpose. In both, the **end-to-end technique** is used, and in both, taping is always done in the direction in which the fascia is more mobile or better able to glide—that way, the recoil of the tape goes in the direction in which the fascia is stuck or restricted. This will help loosen up the restricted area. The difference between these approaches is really only in the application of the tape.

Variation 1: Stretch—Non-Stretch

This variation is aimed at stimulating the fascia with the help of different areas of stretch within the tape strip. You can use "I" tapes, "Y (or V)" tapes, or fan tapes, and cut the tape into the shape and length that suits the target area where you want to apply it.

- Tear the paper backing completely across, and remove around 1–2 inches from one end of the tape strip. As always, this end of the strip—the primary base—should be applied completely without stretch, and then pushed back in a "back-up."

- The primary base should be positioned so it is pointing in the direction where the fascia is stuck and restricted.

- Then peel off the rest of the paper backing, up to a point just before the other end of the tape strip. Hold the tape strip with flat fingers.

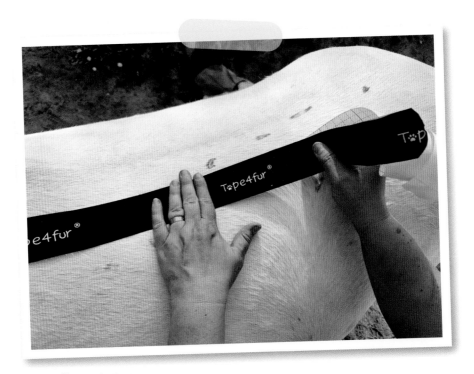

Fig. 11.2: Application of the stretch-free section of a fascia taping (observe that the logo shown here is not stretched!).

- Apply moderate stretch to the tape strip, and then apply about 2 inches of the tape with this stretch in the direction where the fascia is free and mobile.

- Then take the stretch out of the tape (so it does not sag), and apply about 2 inches of tape completely without stretch.

- Then apply another 2 inches of tape with moderate stretch, and another 2 inches without stretch.

- Continue this way until the end of the tape strip, alternating between moderate stretch and no stretch.

- As always, apply the secondary base completely without any stretch, and perform a back-up.

- Rub vigorously but carefully over the entire application to activate the adhesive.

During the application of the tape, always make sure your fingers are flat, so that no uneven or irregular stretching occurs in the tape strip, or in the stretched and unstretched sections!

Depending on the size of the application and the length of the tape strip, you may need to shorten or lengthen the sections of stretch and non-stretch. The shorter the sections, the more you encourage the fascia to move. If the area of concern is rather broad, a "V (or Y)" tape or fan tape can be used. All fingers of these tape cuts have to be applied using the same technique as is described above.

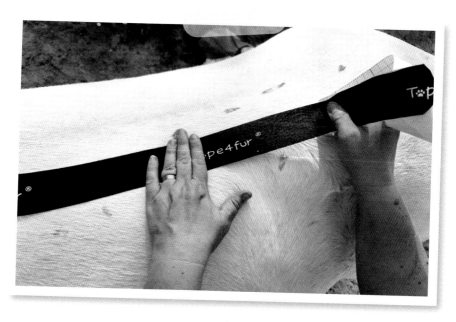

Fig. 11.3: A section with moderate stretch (observe that the logo shown here is visibly distorted by the stretching).

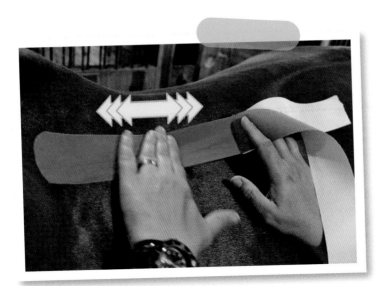

Fig. 11.4: Application of a fascia taping with vibration.

Variation 2: Vibration

In this variation, you will use consistent stretch throughout the tape strip, and the fascia will be manually encouraged to reorganize through vibration.

Pick a tape cut as for the first variation—use whatever is best given the issue you are dealing with and the size of the area of concern.

- Tear the paper backing completely across and remove around 1–2 inches from one end of the tape strip. As always, this end of the strip—the primary base—should be applied completely without stretch, and then pushed back in a "back-up."

- The primary base should be positioned so it is pointing in the direction where the fascia is stuck and restricted.

- Remove the paper backing from the tape, except for the 2 last inches. Hold the tape with flat fingers.

- Apply a mild stretch to the tape strip, and point it in the direction where the fascia is free and mobile.

- With your free hand (in fig. 11.4, the left hand), feel through the tape for the fascia layer, and then start vibrating your hand and fingers against the tape and into this layer as rapidly as you can, stimulating it to reorganize during the tape application.

- Apply the whole tape strip with a mild stretch, vibrating as you go, until about 1–2 inches are left before the secondary base.

- As always, apply the secondary base completely without stretch, and perform a back-up.

- Rub vigorously but carefully over the entire application to activate the adhesive.

This might sound simple at first, but it requires a bit of practice, as you have to coordinate four things at once with only two hands: with one hand, the vibration depth and frequency, and with the other hand, the appropriate stretch for the tape and the alignment of the tape along the body of the horse. On top of that, you have to tape a living creature that may be shifting his weight at that very moment because he wants to scratch his belly.

Fascia taping:

Direction of application: In the direction in which the fascia is freer and more mobile.

Recoil: In the direction in which the fascia is less mobile, stuck, or restricted.

Effect: Release of restricted fascia.

I always recommend trying both varia-tions, and then you can decide for yourself which one suits you better.

Again, if you decide to use a "V (or Y)" tape or fan tape for a broad area of concern, you should use the same approach described above for each finger of the tape cut. This means either all fingers with Variation 1 or all fingers with Variation 2.

Fig. 11.5: A multidirectional fascia taping for the cranial fascia.

More Examples of Fascia Taping

All of the following case studies and taping applications are *supportive* measures intended to complement veterinary, physiotherapeutic, or osteopathic treatments!

Cranial Fascia

This horse presented with constant licking and chewing, and was also sticking her tongue out, even at rest. An examination showed complete restriction of the cranial fasciae in multiple directions, on both sides.

Since the fasciae were tight in a rather large area, and on both sides of her head, I used multiple fan tapes. Variation 1—sections of tape with and without stretch—was used for all of them. Each finger was taped with this variation, always in the direction in which the fascia was free and mobile. The sections of tape with stretch and without stretch were very short (½ inch to an inch) to provide as much stimulation as possible for the cranial fasciae.

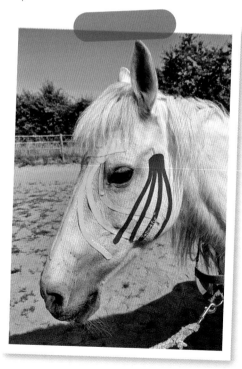

Gluteal Fascia

Although no blockages were present and there were no muscular restrictions, this horse's tail did not swing loosely as it should. The gluteal fasciae were slightly stuck on both sides.

After manual fascia mobilization, I applied the fingers of a fan tape bilaterally with slight stretch under vibration, in order to additionally mobilize the gluteal fascia.

Thoraco-Lumbar Fascia

This horse presented with restriction of the dorsal fascia on the right side over a large area. A fan tape was used, as more surface area could be covered by splitting the tape into fingers. Each finger was applied individually, one after the other, with sections with and without stretch (Variation 1). The thin ends were secured at the level of the scapula with a stretch-free cross anchor to prevent premature detachment.

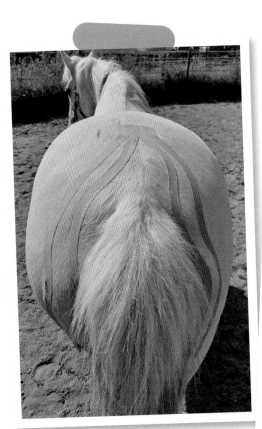

Fig. 11.6: A fascia taping for the gluteal fascia, using a fan tape.

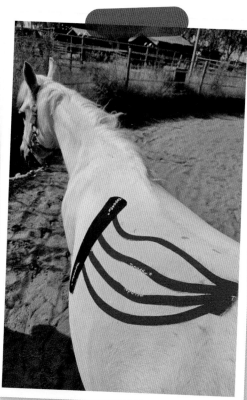

Fig. 11.7: A broad fascia taping for the wide thoracic-lumbar fascia.

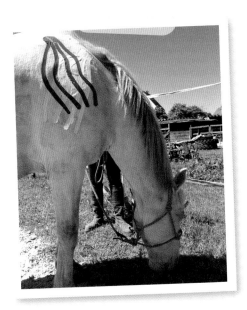

Fig. 11.8: A bidirectional fascia taping for the shoulder fascia.

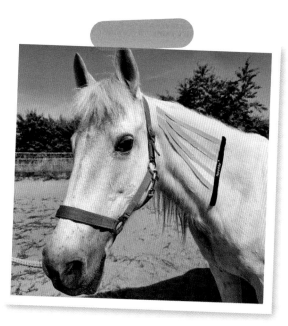

Fig. 11.9: A fascia taping for the neck fascia, with a cross anchor.

Shoulder Fascia

This horse experienced adhesion of her shoulder fascia after a bad fall, which resulted in impact trauma. Her fascia was restricted in several directions. To cover the two most affected directions, I used two fan tapes. Both were taped in the direction that was free to move and glide. I used the vibration technique for both fan tapes; each finger was applied with the same technique.

Neck Fascia

The cause of this horse's trouble was not known for certain, but a bad spill on slippery, frozen ground was suspected. In addition to muscular tension around his poll and upper neck area, as well as blockages in his cervical vertebrae, the left side of his neck fascia was significantly restricted. In addition to massage, manual therapy, and other fascia techniques, a fascia taping was applied to the left side of his neck. Due to the large range of motion in the cervical spine, his neck was pre-stretched as thoroughly as possible to the opposite side while I was applying the tape. The fingers of the fan tape were applied individually, one at a time, using the vibration technique (Variation 2) in the direction in which the fascia was able to move. The ends of the fingers were secured with a stretch-free cross anchor.

Chapter 12

Decompression Taping

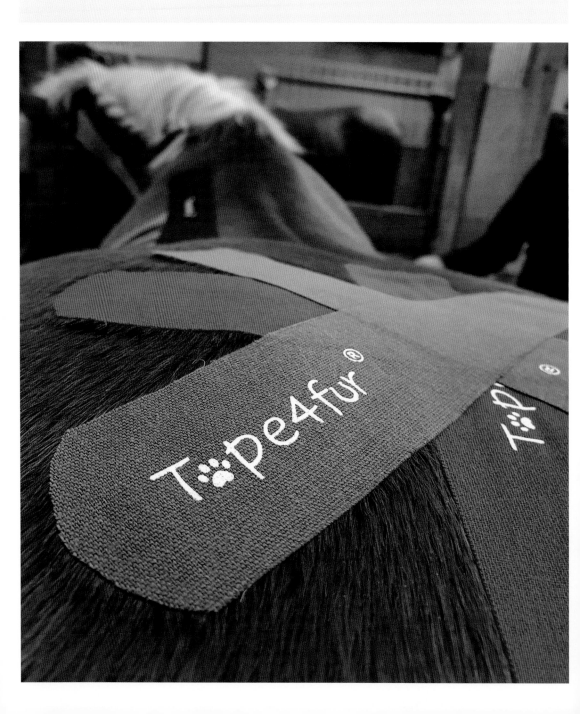

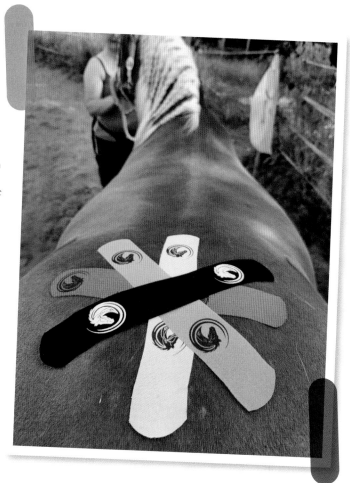

Fig. 12.1: Complete application of a decompression taping for the area of the sacrum and the SI joints.

Uses for Decompression Taping

Whenever there is a very localized problem in the horse, the decompression taping will be your application of choice. Due to its shape and appearance, it is also often called a "star tape" or "flower tape." Other names for this tape are based on its effects: "pain cross" or "space tape." By applying several strips of tape over each other on a certain area, the lifting effect is increased significantly in the center of the application, and it is possible to create a lot of space and greatly reduce compression. This is

the reason for the name "decompression taping." All taping applications have a decom-pressing effect, but that effect is the strongest with this application. The name "space tape," similarly, is applied because this taping increases the amount of space in the decom-pressed tissue the most. This substantial decompression causes the most significant pain-reducing effect kinesiology tape can provide, too, hence the term "pain cross."

It is most often used for the following problems:

- **Trigger points and painful tight spots:** A *trigger point* is an extremely localized tight spot in a muscle. These points can be very painful, and can also lead to secondary pain in neighboring areas of the body. However, painful areas do not necessarily have to have trigger points to be taped with a pain cross.

- **Blockages and misalignments:** When joint blockages—for example, in the lumbar spine or the sacroiliac joints—are resolved, the surrounding soft tissue was usually also affected by the blockage, and may remain very tense and painful. It is always very important to treat the soft tissue, too; otherwise, blockages can recur.

- **Arthritis and arthrosis:** Unfortunately, kinesiology tape does not affect arthritis in and of itself, but it can alleviate the accompanying symptoms, such as pain or swelling. Taping is often used for arthritis in the carpal joint, hip, or hocks, and also for kissing spines, positioned directly over the affected spinal segment.

How to Apply a Decompression Taping

In order to create a symmetrical application that will have the best effect, a decompression taping consists of four "I" tapes of equal length. The length will depend on the area to be taped. For small areas such as the hock, the taping strips can also be split lengthwise, or you can use tape that is 1 inch wide instead of the standard 2 inches. For the temporomandibular joint, you can even split it into fourths. The inside-out technique is always used for a decompression taping, for every tape strip. As an example, here is a detailed step-by-step description for applying a decompression taping over the sacrum and sacroiliac joint area, which is often a problem area for horses and experiences a lot of tension.

- Tear the paper backing across the middle of the first tape strip, and peel it off all but the last 1–2 inches of tape at both ends.

- Hold the tape at both ends with flat fingers, center the strip over the affected area, and apply it with moderate to strong stretch along the

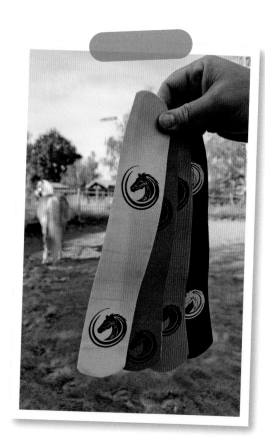

Fig. 12.2: You need four equally long taping strips for a decompression taping.

sacrum (or horizontally, for other areas).

- Remove one end of the paper backing; place this end of the tape backwards on the backs of your fingers, and then apply with absolutely no stretch and do a back-up. Do not remove the paper backing and apply the tape directly, as it will still have the 10 percent pre-stretch it comes with on the paper!

- Rub vigorously but carefully over the tape to activate the adhesive.

- Tear the paper backing of the second tape across the middle, as with the first strip, and remove the paper until just before each end. Hold the tape with flat fingers.

- Center the second tape strip over the affected area at a right angle to the first, and apply with mild to moderate stretch—but with slightly less tension than for the first.

- Apply both ends without any stretch and with back-ups, as previously described.

- Do not forget to rub over the tape strip to activate the adhesive.

- Proceed in the same way with the third and fourth tape strips. Stretch the center of each tape strip from the inside out, hold it with flat fingers, center it over the affected area, and then apply with mild stretch (even milder for the fourth strip—only

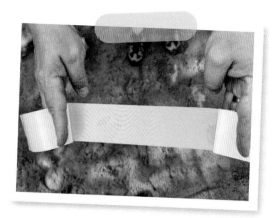

Fig. 12.3: Tear the paper backing across the middle, and remove all but the last 2 inches on both ends. Hold the tape with flat fingers.

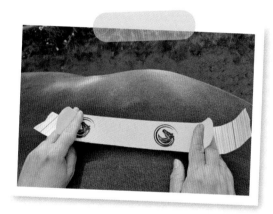

Fig. 12.4: Application of the first tape strip, with flat fingers.

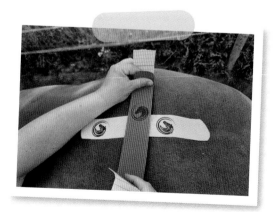

Fig. 12.5: Application of the second tape strip, at a right angle to the first one.

enough so it does not sag). The third strip is positioned diagonally between the first tape strip and one end of the second tape strip; the fourth is positioned diagonally between the first tape strip and the other end of the second.

- The primary and secondary bases should always be applied with no stretch, and you should do a back-up each time. Then rub each tape strip to activate the adhesive.

When applying a decompression taping, make sure, as described above, that you have the most stretch on the first tape strip and then the stretch decreases slightly for each additional "I" tape. In a perfect world, you would apply every tape strip with the exact same amount of stretch, but that is not possible—applying moderate stretch to the fourth tape strip would make it pull on all the tape strips beneath it, and lead to a premature detachment of the entire taping application. So, as described, start with moderate stretch on the first tape strip, and then stretch each subsequent strip less than the previous strip.

When a decompression taping is complete, there are four layers of kinesiology tape over the affected area. Each layer lifts the tissue a little more, so the "lifting effect" is multiplied, and thus this taping maximizes decompression of tissue in the taped area; pressure on tissues and receptions decreases, and pain is reduced.

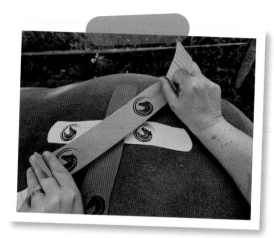

Fig. 12.6: The third tape strip is applied diagonally between the first and one end of the second.

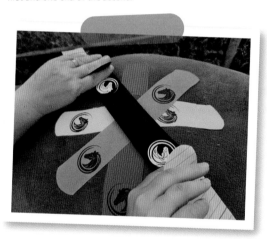

Fig. 12.7: The fourth and last tape strip is applied diagonally also, between the first and the other end of the second; it will end up at a right angle to the third tape strip.

Decompression taping:
Direction of application: From the inside out—from the center of tension outward.
Recoil: From the outside in—toward the center of tension.
Effect: Decompression and relief for tight areas.

More Examples of Decompression Taping

All of the following case studies and taping applications are *supportive* measures intended to complement veterinary, physiotherapeutic, or osteopathic treatments!

Tight Neck and Poll

In the case of tension in the neck area or poll (or both), you can either work with a muscle tape along the straight neck muscle (see the section in chapter 10 on taping the straight neck muscle, page 80) or, if the tension is more localized, you can use a decompression tape, which is what I did for this horse. If the tension is unilateral, you can tape only the affected side; if the issue is bilateral, give each side of the neck its own decompression taping. Since you may not have much area to work with, depending on the part of the neck or poll that is affected, you can cut the tape lengthwise in half, or use tape that is 1 inch wide instead of the standard 2 inches. Mild pre-stretching of the neck to the opposite side is recommended.

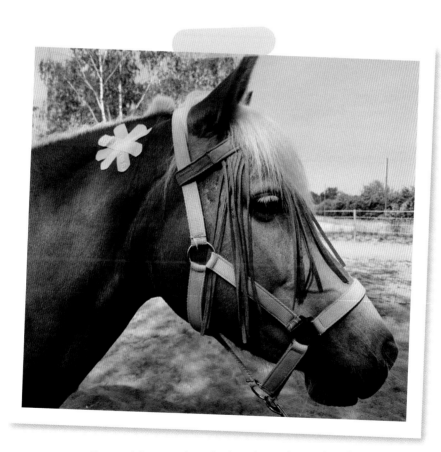

Fig. 12.8: A decompression taping for a trigger point near the poll.

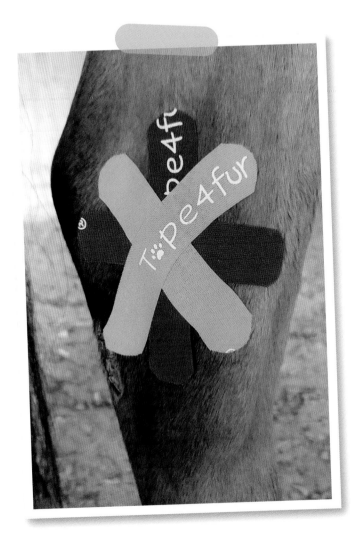

Fig. 12.9: A decompression taping for arthritis in the hock.

Arthritis in the Tarsal Joint and Hock

For osteoarthritis in general, decompression tapes are very, very helpful. Unfortunately, they cannot cure the arthritis itself, but they can help alleviate the accompanying symptoms, including stiffness and pain. In the leg area, it is a good idea to cut 2-inch-wide tape strips lengthwise, or use tape that is already only 1 inch wide, as most horses' legs are quite narrow in this area and a decompression taping using 2-inch-wide tape is simply too large.

In cases involving taping over the hock, I find it works best to apply one decompression taping to the joint medially and one laterally.

In the case of arthritis in the carpal joint, one decompression taping applied cranially, directly on the joint, is usually sufficient (see also fig. 5.1 on page 26).

Painful Bruising after a Fall

As I have mentioned previously, the decompression taping is not nicknamed "the pain cross" for no reason. Since there are four tape strips applied on top of each other over the painful area, the lifting effect is multiplied, and the pain-relieving effect is maximized.

After a fall, the point of this horse's hip and her hip joint were bruised and very painful. Accompanying treatment with a magnetic blanket, a decompression taping was applied to each of the affected areas.

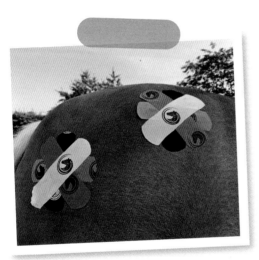

Fig. 12.10: A decompression taping on the point of the hip and the hip joint to reduce pain.

Tight TMJ after Dental Treatment

This horse needed lengthy dental treatments, and his mouth was held open with a mouth gate for extended periods of time. This kind of situation can cause tension or even blockages in the temporomandibular joint, which was exactly what had happened in his case. I applied a decompression taping to the affected joint, as a supportive measure accompanying other treatments. Tape can be cut in half lengthwise, or even in quarters, to allow you to create a decompression taping of the right size for the affected area. In the photo, you can see the decompression taping I applied, combined with a fascia tape—this horse's fascia was also tight and restricted, so I applied both tapings.

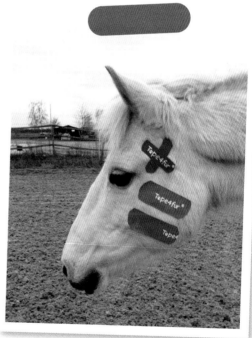

Fig. 12.11: A decompression taping applied to the TMJ, in combination with a fascia taping for the cranial fascia.

Chapter 13

Stabilization Taping

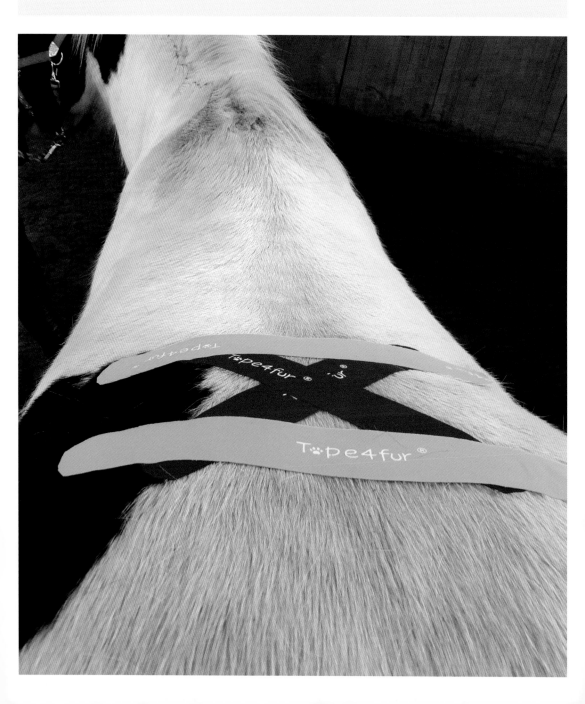

When and Where Is Stabilization Taping Helpful?

There are always horses that are not really suited to being ridden, due to their anatomy and conformation. Horses with extremely long necks and backs fall into this category, especially if they also have a hard time building or maintaining muscles in general or in their necks and backs specifically. Horses with very short backs are also not always the best option for riding horses.

In addition, there are joints and other areas in horses carrying riders that very often must withstand more load than they should, more than they like, or more than is good for them.

These areas include the transition between the thoracic and lumbar spine; the transition from the lumbar spine to the sacrum; the sacroiliac joints; and the neck area, typically from the occipital bone to the first and second cervical vertebra. The transition from cervical to thoracic spine is also often an issue. However, this part of the spine lies so deep under the shoulder blades that it is not easy to affect it with kinesiology tape.

Once blockages in these areas have been resolved, stabilization taping applications can be used to give the affected location even more support and stability, and thereby prevent it from returning to its previous state of blockage as soon as the horse is ridden some more. You can also use stabilization taping preventatively if you know where the horse has a physical weak point—for example, in the case of horses who are characteristically weak in the fetlock or have long pasterns.

How to Apply a Stabilization Taping

In most cases, four "I" tapes are needed for a stabilization taping (exceptions are listed in the examples starting on page 103). The required length depends on the target area. The **inside-out technique** is always used, and **the same level of stretch is maintained throughout**.

As with decompression taping in the previous chapter, tear the paper backing of the "I" tapes across the middle each time; peel off the paper until you are about 2 inches away from the ends, and apply the strip with medium stretch. Apply the ends as usual, without any stretch and with a back-up. Do not forget to use flat fingers!

BUT: With the decompression taping, we applied the effective area of the strip and then let it go in order to then apply the ends. Due to the pre-stretching in the tape, there is a slight recoil at the immediate moment it is let go, until the ends are fully applied.

With a stabilization taping, this recoil should be reduced, and if possible prevented. Therefore, each tape strip is applied with the desired stretch and then held in place with one hand or arm, or held onto by an assistant. The other hand is then used to apply the ends one after the other as usual, completely without any stretch.

Quick Tip: This handling of the tape, holding on to the effective area and simultaneously applying the ends with the other hand, takes some practice. With this application, I like to ask the horse's owners or any riders present

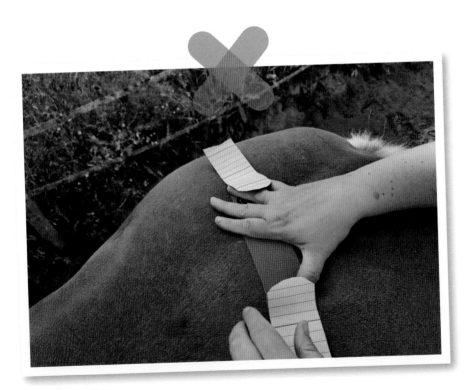

Fig. 13.1: Holding the effective area of the tape in place to prevent recoil.

to help me. I apply the effective area of each tape strip and then have them hold on to it while I apply the ends—without any hassle.

Here is the exact step-by-step procedure, explained here using the sacrum and the sacroiliac joints as an example:

- You need four "I" tapes of equal length with rounded corners.

- Tear the paper backing in the middle of the first tape strip, and remove it up to the last 2 inches of both ends; hold it with flat fingers.

- Center the tape strip over the sacrum at a 45-degree angle.

- Apply the tape with moderate stretch, and then **immediately hold the effective area of the tape strip in place with one hand, or have an assistant hold it. Do not let it recoil.**

- While holding the middle section of the tape like this, remove the paper at one end and apply it as usual, completely without any stretch and with a back-up. Continue holding the effective area in place, and proceed in the same way with the other end.

- Now you or your assistant can let go of the effective area.

- Rub over the tape strip vigorously but carefully to activate the adhesive.

- Apply the second tape strip using exactly the same procedure (holding on to the effective area until the ends are applied without any stretch), but position it at a 45-degree angle in the opposite direction, creating an "X" centered over the area of the sacrum.

- Rub over the second tape strip to activate the adhesive.

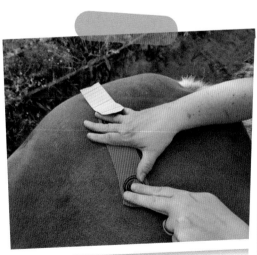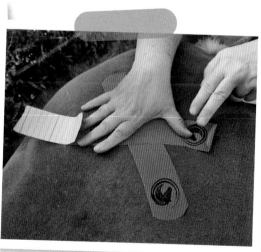

Figs. 13.2 and 13.3: While holding the effective area in place, apply both ends without any stretch.

- Apply the third and fourth strips of tape using the technique described above, too, but center them to the right and left of the sacrum, directly above the sacroiliac joint on each side, and position them parallel to each other.

- Rub over each tape strip individually to activate the adhesive.

To make it easier to see how the pairs of strips are positioned, the "X" in the example (the first and second strips) was taped in blue, and the "I" tapes directly over the sacroiliac joints (the third and fourth strips) were taped in yellow.

By maintaining tension, since you suppressed the immediate recoil of the tape, the "X" stabilizes the sacrum, and the lateral strips provide additional stabilization for the sacroiliac joints.

Quick Tip: For horses that have to travel very, very long distances in a trailer or transporter, stabilization tapes for the sacrum and the sacroiliac joints are a great support option. The horses will be busy balancing themselves all the time during the drive, and this area of the body will have to "work" a lot.

Stabilization taping:
Direction of application: From the inside out, maintaining stretch and suppressing recoil.
Recoil: Sustaining the stretch as described reduces or suppresses recoil.
Effect: The kept tension of the tape supports stability in the area. The cross directly supports the affected area, and the parallel strips support the joint gaps.

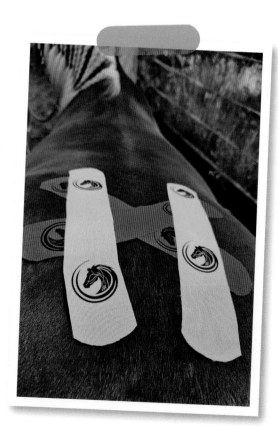

Fig. 13.4: Completed application of a stabilization taping for the sacrum and the sacroiliac joints.

More Examples of Stabilization Taping

All of the following case studies and taping applications are supportive measures intended to complement veterinary, physiotherapeutic, or osteopathic treatments! They can be used in the rehabilitation process, or preventatively in training or to manage known joint weaknesses.

Transition of the Lumbar-Sacral Area

Using the technique described previously, a "cross" was applied directly onto the lumbar-sacral junction of this horse. The pink tape strips in fig. 13.5 are centered directly on this transition area.

In this example, however, the third and fourth tape strips are not aligned over the sacroiliac joints, but rather over the last lumbar vertebra and the cranial edge of the sacrum, in order to additionally stabilize the bones involved in the joint.

All stabilization tapes along the thoracic and lumbar spine follow this basic principle: the "cross" is positioned directly on the affected segment, and one tape strip each goes over the vertebrae involved cranial and caudal of the affected segment (which is to say either side, one on the "horse's head" side of the affected segment, and one on the "horse's tail" side).

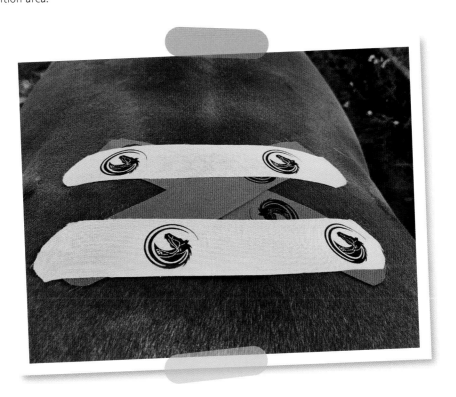

Fig. 13.5: A stabilization taping for the transition between the lumbar spine and the sacrum.

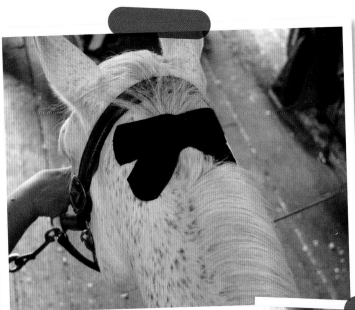

Fig. 13.6: The "cross" of this stabilization taping is positioned over the transition between the first and second cervical vertebrae.

From the Poll to the Second Cervical Vertebra

Using the technique described above, a "cross" is taped over the affected area (here, the first and second cervical vertebrae). Again, two more "I" tapes can then be positioned parallel to the vertebral joint. However, since this area is somewhat smaller than the two previously described examples, I used only one 3-inch-wide "I" tape directly over the joint instead of two parallel tapes.

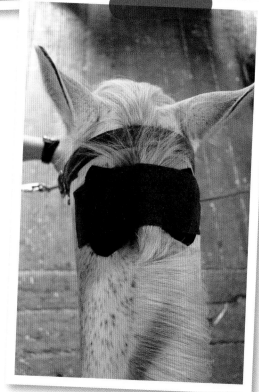

Fig. 13.7. Transverse tape strip of the stabilization taping in the area close to the poll.

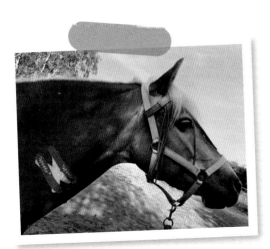

Fig. 13.8. A stabilization taping in the area of the lower neck.

Lower Neck

In the area of the lower cervical spine, stabilization tapes look the same as in the area of the thoracic and lumbar spine. Using the technique described, I applied a "cross" to the affected joint gap of this horse, and one transverse tape to each of the vertebrae cranial and caudal of the affected joint. Since the cervical vertebrae are arranged differently than the thoracic and lumbar vertebrae, due to horse anatomy, I always recommend applying a stabilization taping on each side of the neck. And you should always pre-stretch the neck slightly to the opposite side when you are applying the tape, in order to account for the large range of motion in the neck.

Carpal Joint (Knee)

The carpal joint is one of the previously mentioned exceptions to the usual model of stabilization taping, as there are three joint spaces here, due to the anatomy of the joint and all the small bones present in the knee. All three can be affected by instability or blockage, but they may not all be presenting issues at the same time.

Here, too, I began with the technique described previously, applying a "cross" of two "I" tapes directly onto the cranial area of the carpal joint. I had a helper lift the leg and hold the joint in a slightly flexed position while I taped, so the natural movement of the horse and the bending of the leg during walking would not put too much tension on the tape—this is a good idea whenever you are taping the knees.

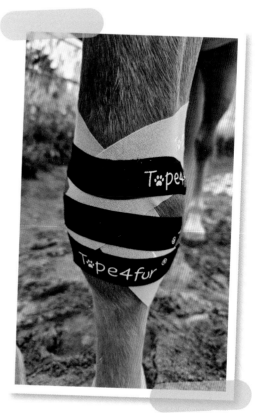

Fig. 13.9: A stabilization taping for the carpal joint and three transverse strips for the joint's gaps.

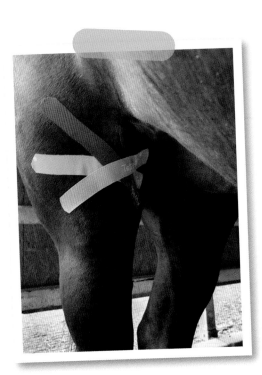

Fig. 13.10: A stabilization taping for the stifle.

Another option for stabilizing the stifle, as well as the entire hind limb, is the stifle sling taping, which is described in detail in chapter 19 (page 142).

Fetlock

A taping application to support the head of the pastern is advisable for horses that are very weak in the fetlock in general, and in the case of diagnosed tendon or suspensory ligament damage, the fetlock should always be supported to further counteract over-stretching of the tendon. Detailed instructions can be found in chapter 16 (page 124), as a fetlock stabilization taping is always the first step before the actual tendon taping.

Stifle

The stifle is also a special case, when it comes to stabilization taping. Only the stifle joint gap is taped. Here, you can see that I used the usual "cross," done in the technique described previously, as well as a single transverse tape strip directly over the joint gap. You must make sure you do not go too far inward with the tape on the inside of the leg, because in this area the skin tends to be very oily and the tape often does not adhere well to it. Always prep the inside of the leg thoroughly with baby powder and a microfiber cloth. Applying transverse tape strips proximal and distal of the stifle gap is suboptimal, as this could restrict the patella in its range of motion and prevent it from sliding the way it needs to.

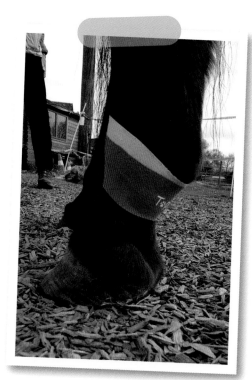

Fig. 13.11: Application of a fetlock stabilization taping.

Tarsal Joint (Hock)

Instability in the hock is common in older horses. This joint can be taped in combination with muscle tapes for the hamstring muscles (see chapter 10, page 60), if they need to be addressed, or on its own for greater stability, as I did for this horse. Using the technique described previously, I applied one "I" tape proximal and distal of the point of the hock (above it and below it, instead of in an "X"

across it) on the back of the leg—the blue and yellow tape strips, in the photo. Then, still using the same technique, I applied one tape strip laterally and medially (along the outside of the leg and then across the inside of the leg) vertically across the tarsal joint. The medial strip is not visible due to the angle of the photo, but runs in the same way as the lateral strip that is shown (the green tape strip).

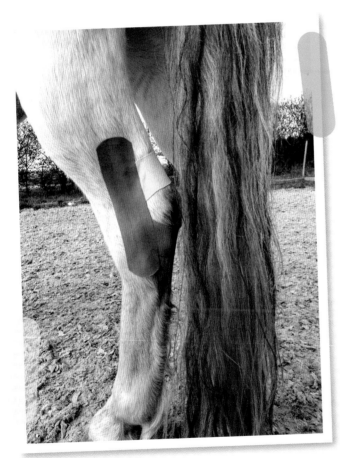

Fig. 13.12: A stabilization taping for the hock.

Chapter 14

Lymph Taping

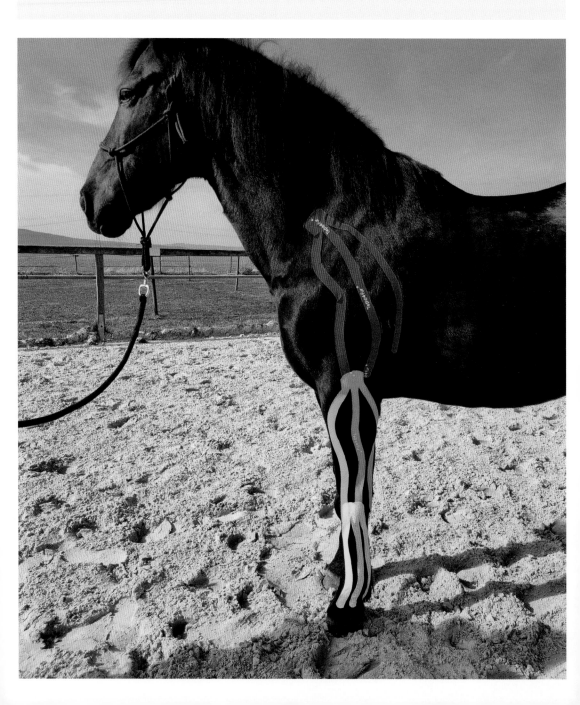

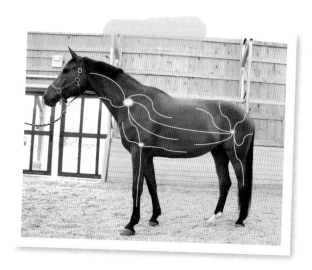

Fig. 14.1: A visualization of the main lymph nodes and their tributary areas in the horse.

Lymph and the Lymphatic System

Lympha is a Latin word meaning "clear water." And that's almost what healthy lymphatic fluid looks like: it is a clear but yellowish fluid, similar to blood plasma and derived from interstitial fluid (the fluid around and between the cells in bodily tissues).

Much like blood, lymph fluid is absorbed from tissue by small, narrow lymph capillaries. These capillaries open into larger lymph vessels that carry lymph to the lymph nodes, which are collection points and filters for lymphatic fluid. From there, lymph is passed on to the neck and shoulder area, where the main jugular lymph node sits; from that node, lymph is then reabsorbed into the bloodstream. Above is a visualization of the most important lymph node areas in horses: the axillary lymph node on the inside of the front leg; the inguinal lymph node on the inside of the hind leg; and the jugular lymph node in front of the shoulder blade. The

lines roughly illustrate the areas of inflow for the respective lymph nodes.

Lymph transports substances that cannot be transported in the bloodstream, and in the lymph nodes, lymph is not just filtered—lymphocytes (white blood cells) are formed and added to it, too. These cells help fight infection and disease, and are an important component of the immune system.

Due to infections, injuries, or sometimes just stall rest, lymphatic fluid may stock up in a horse's extremities. That increased volume and pressure on the lymphatic capillaries can block them so they are no longer able to absorb lymph and carry it out of the legs.

In this case, a lymphatic drainage treatment can help—a special, very gentle form of massage in which the lymphatic system and the main lymph nodes are stimulated to help the lymph disperse. To support lymphatic drainage, you can also apply a lymph taping.

How to Apply a Lymph Taping

The most important tape cut in this case is the fan tape; fan tapes can be used to create a "lymphatic row" or "lymphatic grid," depending on which is necessary and the degree of swelling. A fan tape consists of a closed end, the primary base, with the rest of the tape strip cut into three to five "fingers" (see the section on fan tapes in chapter 8, starting on page 43). I recommend that you consider using a wider kind of kinesiology tape—3 inches wide, instead of the standard 2 inches—for lymph tapings, because you can cut more fingers from wider pieces of tape, and can cover the target area more effectively.

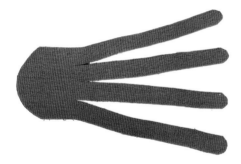

Fig. 14.2: Fan tapes are always used for lymph taping applications.

Lymph tapings use the **end-to-end technique**. Always start with the closed primary base, applied on or close to a lymph node, and then apply the fingers, directed distally toward the swelling—toward the leg. This aligns the recoil in the tape toward the primary base, in the direction of the lymph node, thus directing the drainage of the stocked-up fluid up toward the node and out of the leg.

Here is the general procedure for a lymph taping:

- Cut three to four fan tapes with relatively long fingers—the number you should use depends on the height of the swelling on the leg, as well as the size of the swelling and the size of the horse.

- Tear the paper backing on all of your fan tapes at the transition from the primary base to the tape "fingers," and fold over the edge of it (see fig. 14.3). This will help you get a better grip on the paper backing for each finger during application.

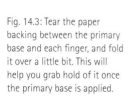

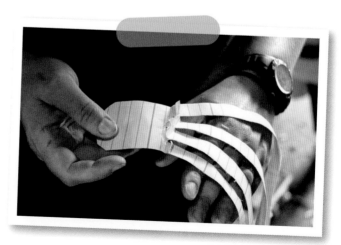

Fig. 14.3: Tear the paper backing between the primary base and each finger, and fold it over a little bit. This will help you grab hold of it once the primary base is applied.

- If the swelling is on the forehand, ask a helper to stretch the horse's neck away from you while you are applying the first fan tape. This will prevent the primary base from overstretching and detaching prematurely, should the horse turn his head and neck to that side. This is not necessary for the hindquarters, where the range of motion is smaller than that of the neck and forehand.

- Remove the paper backing from the primary base of the fan tape. Center this over the jugular lymph node of the forehand, or the inguinal lymph node on the hindquarters, and apply it without any stretch.

- When you apply the fingers, use the stretch the tape comes off the paper with, that 10 percent pre-stretch that is already present. Directly apply each finger while pulling off the paper (see fig. 11.4).

- Apply the fingers of the fan tape one after the other, directing them toward the swollen limb or other area of swelling, spreading them out over as large an area as possible in a straight or wavy line. The wavy line is often the better option, as it increases the coverage of the taping application even further.

- As always, the ends of the tape fingers are applied without any stretch.

- After applying all the tape fingers of the fan tape, rub very carefully over each of them to activate the adhesive.

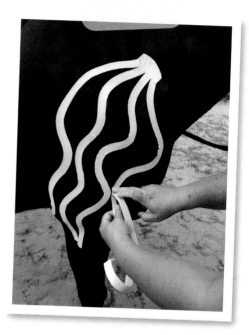

Fig. 14.4: The fingers of this fan tape are applied directly as the paper backing is removed, using the tape's 10 percent pre-stretch. This is also called the "off-paper stretch."

Lymph taping:
Direction of application: From the lymph node toward the swelling.
Recoil: From the swelling toward the lymph node.
Effect: Supporting transportation of stocked-up fluid out of the extremities.

Be careful with the thin tape fingers! It is best to always rub from the base toward the ends of the fingers, not vice versa, so as not to accidentally rub the thin finger ends right off the hair.

The Lymph Row

If the horse has an extremity, whether fore or hind, that is completely swollen and stocked up, you should connect the fan tapes along this swelling to form a "lymph row."

Always start close to the body, at the biggest lymph node, and tape toward the swelling. A stocked-up limb is similar to a traffic jam: you have to break it up by creating space for the cars at the front of the jam—the lymph fluid right at the edge of the swelling—to drive away, and then the cars trapped behind them will be able to follow and drive away, too.

- The first fan tape is applied as described above.

- The base of the second fan tape is applied without any stretch, positioned so it overlaps at least one of the ends of the fingers of the primary fan tape, so together they will form a continuous "row" of tape, to provide a clear path for the lymph to follow to leave the swollen limb (see fig. 14.6).

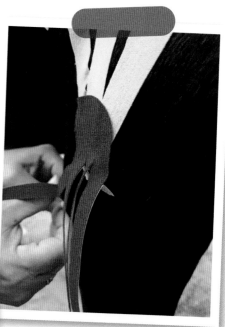

Fig. 14.6: The base of the second fan tape is applied so that it overlaps the finger ends of the previous fan tape to create a continuous path for the lymph to follow.

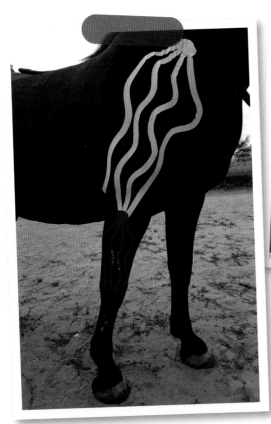

Fig. 14.5: A "lymph row" on the front leg, reaching from the jugular lymph node to the highest part of the swelling on the leg.

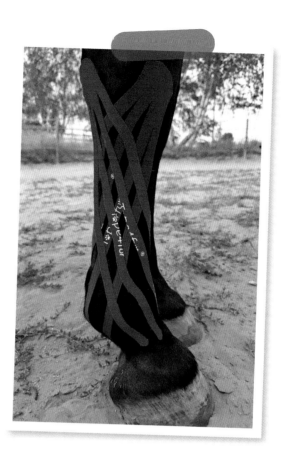

Fig. 14.7: A "lymph grid" around the lower leg.

- Proceed in the same way with the third fan tape: apply a stretch-free base in a position where it overlaps one or several finger ends from the previous fan tape. Continue working distally, toward the swelling, until the swelling is completely covered.

- It is better to string several fan tapes together than to use one very long fan tape. Since you are only using the 10 percent "off-paper" stretch in the tape, you do not have a lot of recoil, and some of the recoil will get lost if you are using very long tape fingers.

The Lymph Grid

If there is swelling in the lower part of the limb only, and the upper part of the leg is not swollen, which means the lymph flow in that area is still functional, the "lymph grid" should be your lymph taping application of choice.

- Apply two to four fan tapes using the technique described at the beginning of this chapter (page 110).

- The bases of the fan tapes should all be positioned at the same height, but at different points around the leg, just above the swelling. All tape fingers should be applied reaching distally toward the swelling. Tape

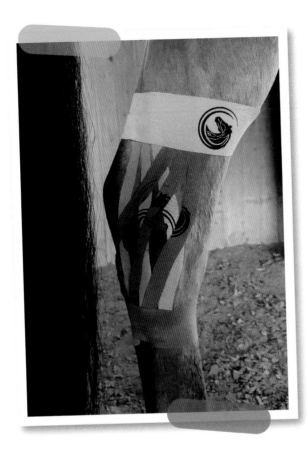

Fig. 14.8: A lymph grid on the inside of the hock, where the swelling was located, with two anchors to secure the lymph taping.

them in an overlapping, staggered fashion, such that they form a grid pattern that covers the swelling completely.

- The bases of the tapes should also point in the direction of the lymph nodes, but all at different angles. For example, one starts on the front of the leg, with the fingers running diagonally across the medial or lateral side of the leg. Another tape may start medially, slanting cranially or caudally. Likewise, a fan tape can start on the outside of the leg or the back of the leg, and slant forward.

You can also combine a lymph row with this lymph grid setup. Apply the lymph row from proximal to distal, and then arrange several more fan tapes in a lymph grid on the lower part of the limb. Whether you use this arrangement depends entirely on the situation and swelling, and your preferences as a therapist.

Generally, when you are applying a lymph taping, I recommend you secure the many thin finger ends with one or more anchors. These are "I" tapes that are applied completely without stretch. They are used to protect the actual application and help it stick longer, and should not otherwise influence it—that's why it is so important for these anchors to be stretch-free! You can apply the anchors either once around the limb, or only in the area of the finger ends, thereby covering as many of them as possible.

Always make sure your fan tapes run from proximal (close to the body) to distal (toward the end of the limb), since this is how lymphatic vessels run. I often see pictures of lymph tapings applied horizontally. Since lymph vessels do not run horizontally, this arrangement does not make much sense!

BE AWARE: With many lymph tapings, a clear reduction in swelling can be seen within just 24 hours. The application is usually no longer under tension at that point, because the volume of the swelling has been reduced, which means the kinesiology tape is typically sagging. At that point, the tape can be removed; it has done its job, and once it is no longer stretched, it has little to no influence on lymph flow anyway. If you feel it is necessary, you can apply a new lymph taping, which is applied to the remaining swelling at its current size and shape and will therefore have a meaningful amount of stretch again.

More Examples of Lymph Taping

All of the following case studies and taping applications are supportive measures intended to complement veterinary, physiotherapeutic, or osteopathic treatments!

Swelling after Acute Injury Following a Kick to the Lower Leg

After an injury from a kick, which left a 2-inch abrasion on this horse's cannon bone, there was an approximately palm-sized swelling around the abrasion on the following day. The swelling was not warm to the touch; since there was no heat or inflammatory process occurring, and it was only a small swelling on

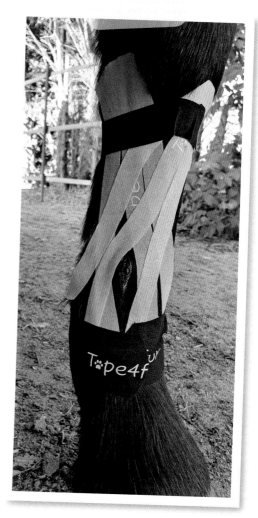

Fig. 14.9: A lymph taping for the lower extremity, after injury from a kick.

the upper front cannon bone, I applied a lymph grid taping with two fan tapes. One was applied medially, and one laterally, so the fingers crossed over the swelling on the front of the cannon bone. The actual wound site was not taped over.

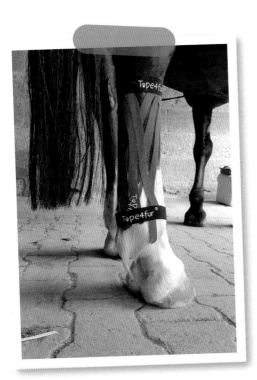

Fig. 14.10: A lymph taping on the lower extremity to address chronic swelling around the fetlock.

Chronic Swelling after Surgery on the Annular Ligament

After successful surgery on his annular ligament several years ago, this horse presented with an area around the fetlock that stocked up every now and then. Following other lymphatic drainage treatment, a lymph taping in the form of a lymph grid was applied to the caudal area of her cannon bone and fetlock. One fan tape was applied medially and one laterally, so the ends of the fingers crossed at the back of the fetlock. In addition, the whole application was secured with anchors, since this horse also liked to scratch himself in that area, and the tape was thus secured.

Osteoarthritis of the Hock with Surrounding Swelling

This horse had a known spavin condition and osteoarthritis in the hock of his right hind for several years. Depending on the weather conditions and also his workload, the area around and above the hock stocked up every now and then.

I applied a lymph row taping, starting at the main lymph node of the hindquarters. Two more tapes were applied at the level of the stifle, overlapping with the first tape to extend the row. One of them ran laterally, and one ran to the medial side of the hock. The ends of the fingers were secured with an anchor, and the transition from the first fan tape to the two subsequent fan tapes was also secured with a transverse anchor.

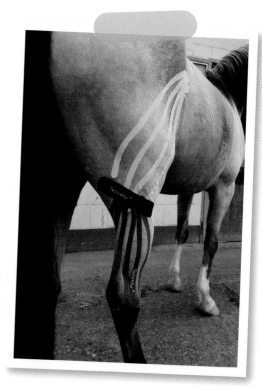

Fig. 14.11: A lymph taping on the hind leg for swelling due to osteoarthritis in the hock.

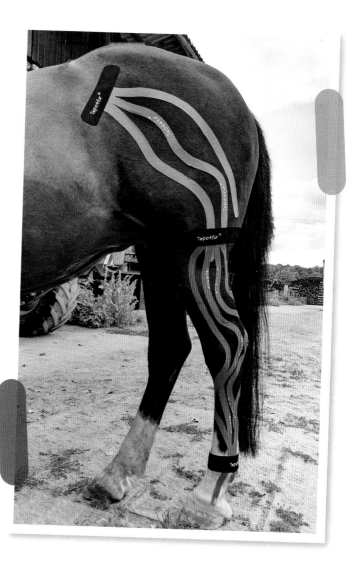

Fig. 14.12: A lymph taping for the whole hind leg.

Chronic Swelling after Inflammatory Process in the Hock

This horse had an inflammatory process in her hock, which was treated by her veterinarian. However, a residual swelling remained, which extended from the hock down all the way to the fetlock.

I applied a lymph row along the entire limb, starting at the level of the inguinal lymph node. Above the hock, running laterally and starting at the hock, the second and third tapes were applied, medial and lateral, running all the way to the fetlock. Here, too, several stretch-free transverse anchors were included to protect the application.

Chapter 15

Hematoma Taping

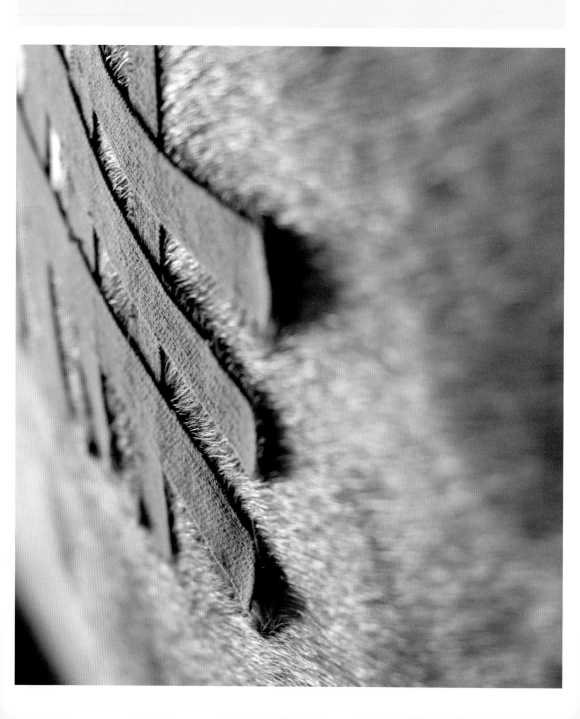

Everyone has probably had a hematoma—the clinical term for a bruise—at some point in their life. Bang your shins or your elbow, and there is a big bruise on the spot in no time. This also happens to our horses thanks to kicks, falls, or even insect bites. Often, hematomas in horses go by unnoticed, because you can't see the bruise through the coat covering the horse's skin, and if the swelling that accompanies it is very small, you may not feel it, either. Larger areas of swelling are more noticeable.

A hematoma is caused by a local hemorrhage; the pressure on and around the area is increased, drainage of metabolic waste products is disturbed, and fluid stocks up locally, which is why the whole thing can be quite painful. A hematoma taping can help.

Hematoma tapings are always applied to local swellings on the body; the lymph tapings from the previous chapter, by contrast, are used to address swellings in the limbs.

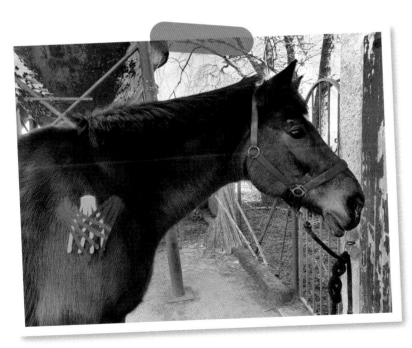

Fig. 15.1: A completed hematoma taping application on the shoulder area.

How to Apply a Hematoma Taping

Much like a lymph taping, a hematoma taping usually uses a fan tape with a closed base and three to five fingers. Depending on the size of the hematoma, you may want to use tape that is 3 inches wide instead of the standard 2 inches wide, in order to cover a larger area. As described in the previous chapter, after cutting your fan tape, tear the paper across the back and fold the edges of the tear over at the transitions between the base and the fingers. That way, you can find the folded edge quickly and easily, and pull the paper off one finger at a time during application. As with all fan tapes, this taping uses the **end-to-end technique**.

As always, adjust the length and number of tapes you use to suit the size of the area of concern—in this case, the hematoma. With hematoma tapes, this saying applies: The more, the better. The more fan tapes you apply, the more thoroughly and rapidly you stimulate drainage of stocked-up fluids. The base of the fan tape should point away from the center of the swelling, and the fingers should be applied running toward the swelling, covering it completely.

- Remove the paper backing from the base of the first fan tape, and apply this primary base near but not on the swelling, without any stretch.

- Take one of the two outermost tape fingers, and apply it along the corresponding outer edge of the swelling with no more than that mild 10 percent pre-stretch it has as it comes off the paper. Simply pull the paper backing off gently, applying the tape finger as you go.

- Apply the other outermost tape finger along the other outer edge of the swelling, using the off-paper stretch. Now the hematoma is "outlined" on both sides.

- Apply the remaining tape fingers evenly over the swelling. Again, use only the stretch the tape already has in it as it comes off its paper backing.

- Make sure the ends of the fingers are always applied without any stretch.

- Rub over each portion of the tape to activate the adhesive. As for the lymph taping applications, remember to rub from the tape base toward the ends of the tape fingers and not the

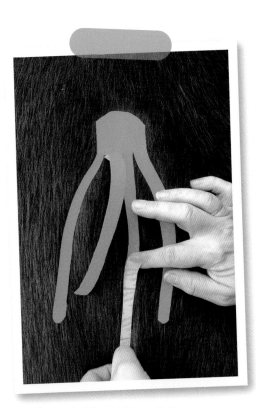

Fig. 15.2: Applying the fingers of a fan tape using the 10 percent off-paper stretch.

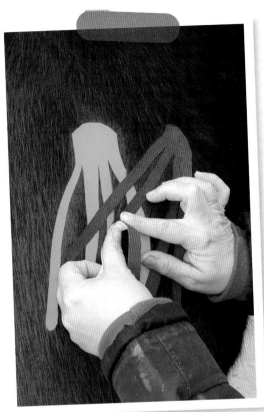

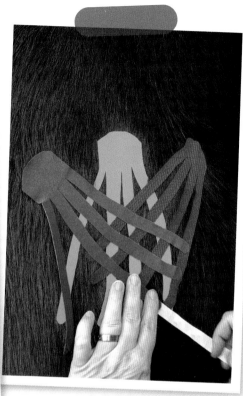

Figs. 15.3 and 15.4: Various fan tapes applied in multiple directions.

other way around, to avoid a situation where the motion of rubbing pulls those thin, narrow tape fingers off right after you applied them.

Additional fan tapes are applied in the same way; each of their bases should point in a different direction. This promotes and accelerates outflow of stocked-up metabolic waste products in multiple directions. The more drainage directions, the better.

BE AWARE: As long as the swelling you are addressing is on the trunk, your fan tapes can point in all directions, as in the example here. However, if the swelling is directly above a leg, or even on the upper part of the leg, DO

NOT apply any fan tapes with the base pointing downward toward the leg. This will only serve to stimulate drainage down into the leg instead of up out of it, which means fluid may simply start stocking up again farther down the leg.

> **Hematoma taping:**
> **Direction of application:** Toward the swelling.
> **Recoil:** Away from the swelling.
> **Effect:** Stimulation of drainage for stocked-up fluid.

More Examples of Hematoma Taping

All of the following case studies and taping applications are *supportive* measures intended to complement veterinary, physiotherapeutic, or osteopathic treatments!

Swelling on the Belly after a Bite from Another Horse

After this horse was bitten by another horse, a palm-sized swelling developed diagonally next to the actual bite wound. I applied three fan tapes around the swelling. Each of the tape bases pointed in different directions away from the swelling, in order to stimulate drainage over a larger area. No tape was applied in the direction of the actual bite wound, as the injury was not yet completely healed and had not closed on the surface.

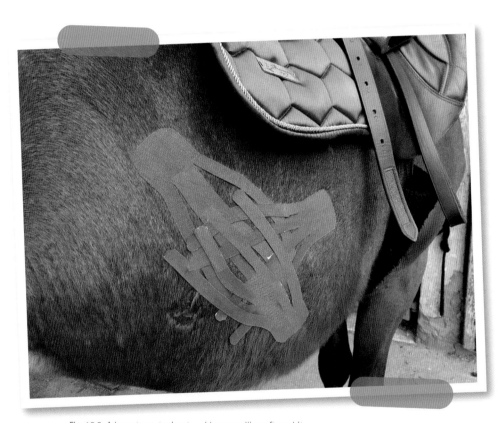

Fig. 15.5: A hematoma taping to address swelling after a bite.

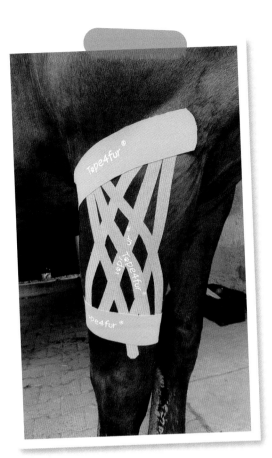

Fig. 15.6: A hematoma taping on the front leg to address a bruise.

Bruise on Front Leg with Swelling after a Fall

This horse was romping around in her paddock and fell, hitting the upper part of her foreleg on the only large stone present. The lateral side of the leg was swollen in spots. I applied two fan tapes with the bases pointing in the direction of the center of the body in order to prevent accumulated fluid from flowing downwards and possibly stocking up in her leg.

The whole application was secured proximally and distally with completely stretch-free cross anchors.

Swelling after an Insect Bite

This horse's insect bite had become infected, and there was severe swelling and thickness directly around the puncture site. After the primary inflammatory process had subsided and the wound area was no longer "hot," swelling remained. Since the insect bite was still open, I had to tape around it.

Three "V (or Y)" tapes were applied around the puncture site. The bases pointed away from the swelling to stimulate drainage in these directions.

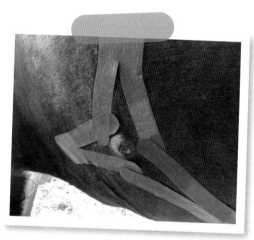

Fig. 15.7: A hematoma taping around an insect bite.

Chapter 16

Tendon Taping

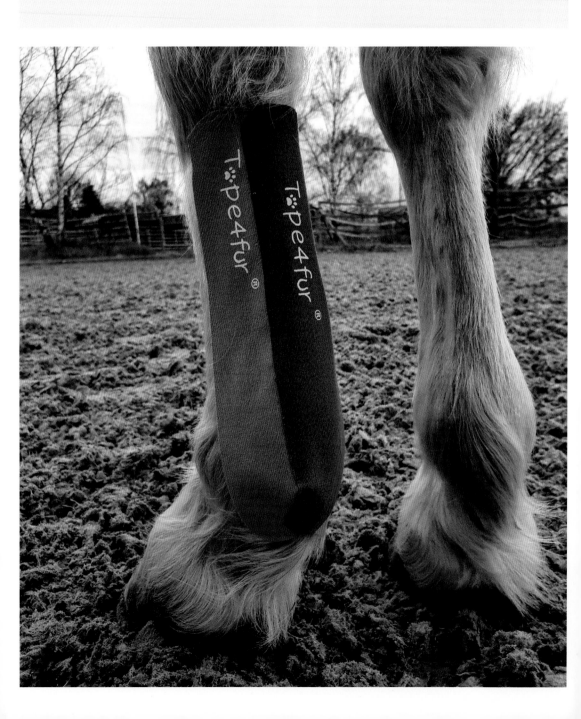

The Tendons

As already explained in chapter 10 (page 60), muscles are attached to bones at their origin and their insertion via tendons. Chapter 9 (page 54) explained that muscles and their muscle fibers are surrounded by fascia. The parallel fibrous tendons, which look like whitish strands, are derived from these connective tissue fasciae sheaths.

Tendons contain very few elastic fibers, which makes them very resistant to stretching and tearing. However, long tendons such as the superficial and deep flexor tendons can have a certain elasticity and springiness because of their length. This allows, for example, the suspensory ligament that supports the fetlock to touch the ground under extreme load, such as during the landing after a jump.

When a horse has weak fetlocks or has sustained injuries to his flexor tendons, the tendon taping can be used. It can also be used to address abnormal tendon position and tendon shortening.

Tendon tapings are mostly used in rehabilitation, but they also have preventive applications in training, as it is quite useful to be able to give tendons more support and stability.

How to Apply a Tendon Taping

Fetlock Support and Stabilization Taping
The first step in every tendon taping is the fetlock support taping. This is always applied before the actual tendon taping, regardless of whether the tendon being addressed is the deep or superficial flexor tendon or the suspensory ligament.

Since almost all tendon damage is caused by overuse and overstretching, it is important to support the fetlock, as this counteracts further overstretching. A fetlock support taping is also excellent as a preventive measure applied in advance of daily training.

For a fetlock support taping, two "I" tapes of equal length with rounded corners are needed. These should be measured to a length that will let them lie around the fetlock joint at the same angle as that at which the fetlock joint is positioned. The inside-out technique is used with steady stretch, as with the stabilization tapings in chapter 13 (page 98).

- Tear the paper backing of the first tape strip across the middle. Only expose a maximum of 4 inches of tape!

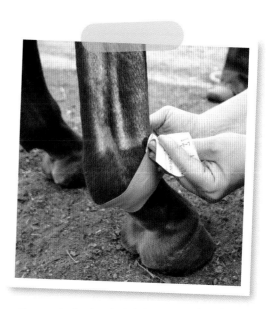

Fig. 16.1: Application of a fetlock support taping using steady stretch, below the fetlock.

- Grasp the tape on the right and left around the back of the fetlock and apply these 4 inches with moderate stretch below the fetlock, following the angle of the joint diagonally upwards.

- As with a stabilization taping, hold this applied area of the tape in place with your free hand (or have a helper hold onto it) to prevent recoil.

- With the other hand, remove the rest of the paper backing from one end of the tape strip, and apply it forward and upward around the fetlock with only off-paper stretch. The last inch should be applied without any stretch at all.

- Do the same with the second end. The stretch-free ends can overlap.

- When both ends are applied, you can let go of the middle section.

- Rub vigorously but carefully over the tape strip to activate the adhesive.

- Apply the second tape strip the same way: tear the backing across the middle, remove about 4 inches of paper, and apply the tape with moderate stretch below the fetlock, applying the ends with no stretch.

- **BUT** the second tape strip is applied a little lower, and angled a little more flatly. This gives the fetlock support from two angles.

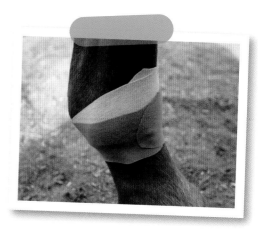

Fig. 16.2: Completed application of a fetlock support and stabilization taping, with two tape strips applied at different angles.

Fetlock support taping:
Direction of application: From the inside out, maintaining stretch.
Recoil: No recoil, since stretch is maintained.
Effect: Stabilization of the fetlock by maintaining stretch and suppressing recoil.

Tendon Taping

Using the deep flexor tendon of a foreleg as an example, I will explain the actual application for the tendon step by step. Here, too, it is important to counteract any further over-stretching of an injured or torn tendon. **The application is completely identical if done on the hind leg.**

For the deep flexor tendon, two "I" tapes of equal length are needed, measured from below the carpal joint to below the fetlock joint. The **end-to-end technique** is used.

- The first "I" tape is applied laterally.

- Remove approximately 1 inch of the paper backing from one end of the tape strip.

- Apply this end, the primary base, without any stretch, directly below the carpal joint and running parallel to the caudal edge of the cannon bone.

- Remove the remaining paper except for the last inch. Hold the tape with flat fingers and apply the effective area with mild stretch, directed distally along the caudal edge of the cannon bone, running toward the fetlock.

- Apply the secondary base below the fetlock, completely without stretch

- Rub vigorously but carefully over the tape strip to activate the adhesive.

- The second tape strip is applied medially on the leg, in identical alignment. These two tape strips may overlap below the fetlock.

- Rub vigorously but carefully over the second tape strip to activate the adhesive.

It is a good idea to secure this taping application with stretch-free cross anchors at the proximal and distal ends, as horses often like to rub their heads against their legs in this area, which could loosen the taping application and cause premature detachment.

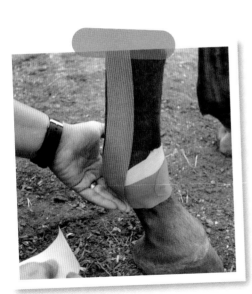

Fig. 16.3: Application of the lateral "I" tape for a deep flexor tendon taping, from the carpal joint toward the fetlock.

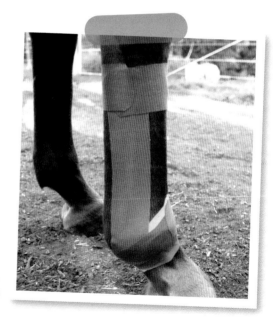

Fig. 16.4: Completed application of a tendon taping for the deep flexor tendon, with stretch-free cross-anchors below the carpal joint and below the fetlock.

BE AWARE: The direction of the application described above—running from the carpal joint to the fetlock—is used to address injuries and overstretching of the tendon.

Tendon taping for injuries, tears, and overstretching:
Direction of application: From the carpal or tarsal joint down to the fetlock.
Recoil: From the fetlock up toward the carpal or tarsal joint.
Effect: Stimulating contraction of the tendon, counteracting any further overstretching.

If there is a congenital or chronic shortening of the tendon, however, such as that associated with a club foot or with abnormal tendon position, you do not want to promote shortening. On the contrary, in this case you will be taping to stimulate stretching of the shortened tendon, and so the direction of the application must be reversed: tape upward from the fetlock to the carpal or tarsal joint in order to support elongation of the tendon with the recoil of the tape. You also do not necessarily need a fetlock support tape first, for this kind of taping.

Tendon taping for abnormal position or congenital conditions accompanied by shortening of the tendon:
Direction of application: From the fetlock upward to the carpal or tarsal joint.
Recoil: From the carpal or tarsal joint down toward the fetlock.
Effect: Stimulating elongation of the shortened tendon.

More Examples of Tendon Taping

Superficial Flexor Tendon

Depending on the width of the horse's leg and his tendon, a wider tape may be a good choice here to better cover the superficial flexor tendon.

For the superficial flexor tendon, start in the same way as described previously, with a fetlock support taping. Instead of the two taping strips running medially and laterally along the deep flexor tendon, only one "I" tape is applied over the back of the leg, following the superficial flexor tendon from proximal to distal—from below the carpal or tarsal joint down to below the fetlock. Apply this "I" tape with very little stretch to prevent bowing of the superficial flexor tendon. Again, stretch-free cross anchors positioned proximally and distally at the ends of the tendon tape are a good idea.

This taping applies as previously described to a situation of tendon overstretching, strain, or injury. If the issue is instead tendon shortening, then, again, the direction of taping should be reversed, with the application taped from a

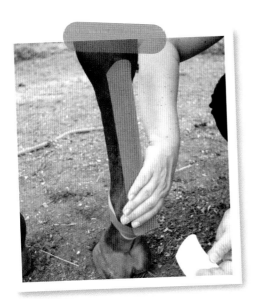

Fig. 16.5: Application of a tendon taping for the superficial flexor tendon.

under the fetlock the same way, and crosses over to the lateral side. Thus, they both cross underneath the fetlock to the opposite side. The secondary bases of the "I" tapes can be applied to the hoof, without any stretch.

This approach not only best covers the suspensory ligament, it also gives additional support to the fetlock because the tape strips cross over underneath it.

Here, I usually just use one stretch-free cross anchor at the proximal end of the taping application, just below the carpal or tarsal joint. Kinesiology tape adheres extremely well to the hoof, so no additional anchor is needed there. The hoof must be clean and dry before application!

distal position to a proximal position—from the fetlock up to the carpal or tarsal joint.

Suspensory Ligament

If the suspensory ligament is the area of concern, start with a fetlock support taping as the first step. As with the deep flexor tendon, one "I" tape is then taped medially, and one laterally. However, since the suspensory ligament splits into two branches below the fetlock, which then run forward and downward to the right and left of the fetlock, toward the hoof, the "I" tapes you use should be significantly longer here than for a deep flexor tendon taping. To avoid kinking the tape at the level of the fetlock, I cross the lateral tape strip under the fetlock and over to the medial side, and then, following the suspensory ligament, bring it forward and downward toward the hoof. The medial tape strip is then guided

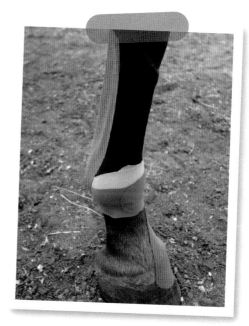

Fig. 16.6: A taping application for support of the suspensory ligament. The first "I" tape is positioned medially, along the caudal edge of the cannon bone, crossing over under the fetlock to the opposite side and angling forward and downward toward the hoof. A second identical strip is applied on the opposite side.

Chapter 17

Scar Taping

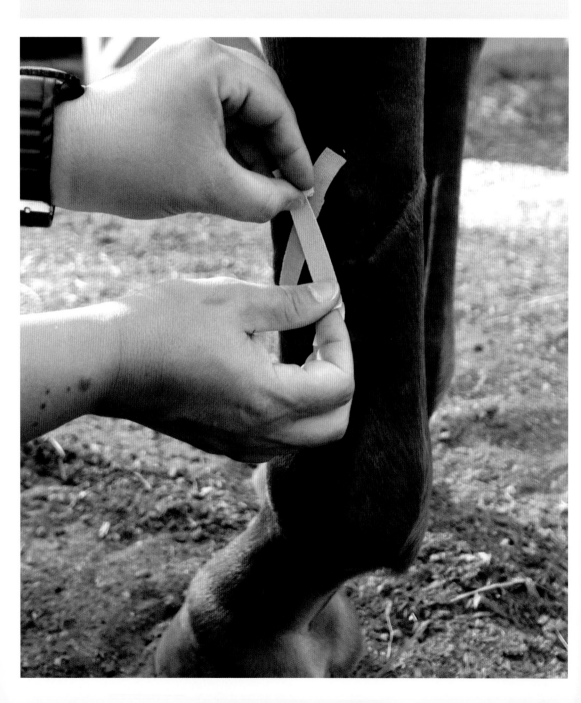

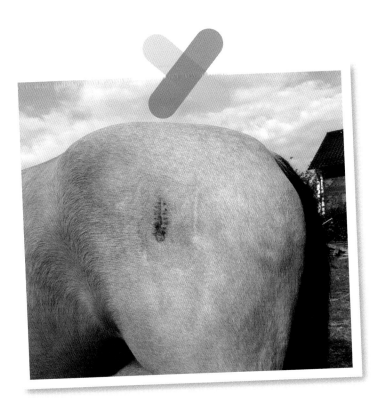

Fig. 17.1: A sutured scar on the flank after this horse injured himself on a paddock post.

Scar Tissue

Scar tissue is formed when deeper layers of the skin are injured, either by a wound or during a needed surgical operation. Unfortunately, the body is not able to repair or reproduce damaged or destroyed skin structure perfectly. Instead, lost tissue is replaced with fibrous connective tissue. When it appears in uninjured parts of the body, functioning normally, the fibers in this kind of connective tissue are arranged parallel to each other. Unfortunately, this is not the case when this connective tissue is used to create a scar. The fibers in scar tissue are arranged in an irregular, crisscross pattern, and grow to meet the existing tissue around the injured area in a haphazard, disorganized manner. As a result, some of the features of normal, uninjured skin, such as hair, sebaceous glands, and sweat glands, that have been destroyed in these areas can no longer grow back as they were before. Regular skin function is often compromised in scar tissue.

Sometimes the connective tissue that forms a scar is overproduced by the body in error; this can cause scar proliferation or scar bulges. By contrast, if scar tissue is underproduced and there is not enough connective tissue forming, the scar will appear sunken or retracted.

The most important point is that the connective tissue in a scar is much less elastic than the skin it is replacing, due to the irregular way its fibers grow. If a scar is located on an area that is under a lot of stress, such as over a joint, it can restrict movement.

The goal of scar treatment and scar massage is to make this tissue softer and more elastic, and to stimulate circulation. Scar taping is very helpful to support this kind of treatment.

How to Apply a Scar Taping

Cut many small strips of tape, matching the size and length of the scar. In this one single instance, it is not necessary to round the corners of these strips. Do, however, make sure that all the strips are cut lengthwise, not across the width of the tape roll; kinesiology tape does not stretch across its width, so you will not be able to apply stretch to the tape if you cut it this way.

Use the **inside-out technique**. Tear the paper backing of the strips across the middle, and stretch the tape from the center to the ends. This creates recoil toward the center of the tape strip—which means toward the scar, once the tape is applied.

- Tear the paper backing of the first small tape strip across the middle,

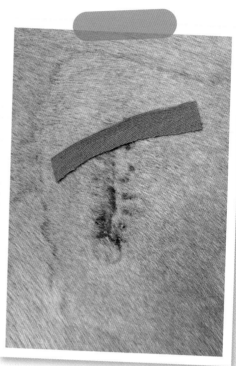

Fig. 17.3: The first "I" tape is applied at a 30–45 degree angle relative to the scar, using the inside-out technique.

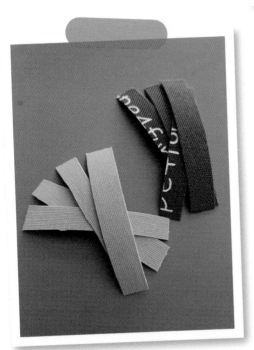

Fig. 17.2: A lot of very small "I" tapes are needed for a scar taping.

and remove it on both sides until just before the ends.

- Apply the tape with medium stretch from the inside to the outside, positioned at an angle of 30–45 degrees relative to the scar. Apply both ends without any stretch, as usual.

- Apply the second small tape strip in the same way. Tear the paper across the middle, remove it until just before the ends, and then apply the effective area of the strip with medium stretch and the ends without any stretch. **But this time, position it at a 30–45 degree angle relative to the scar in the other**

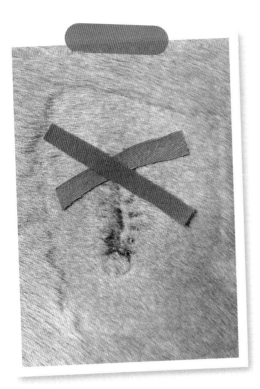

Fig. 17.4: The second tape strip, applied at a 30–45 degree angle relative to the scar but in the opposite direction.

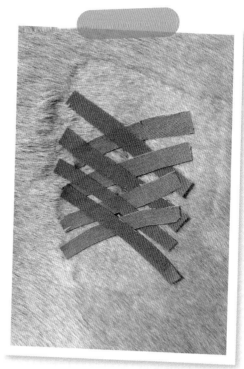

Fig. 17.5: A complete scar taping application that looks like a section of chain-link fence.

direction. The first two strips of tape will thus form a small cross.

- Continuing to use the inside-out technique, apply the third small strip in the same way, parallel to the first tape strip, and the fourth strip likewise, parallel to the second strip.

- Keep on going in the same way. The fifth strip should be applied parallel to the first and third strips, and the sixth strip parallel to the second and fourth, and so on.

- You will line up the tape strips one cross at a time along the scar, so that at the end the application looks almost like a section of chain-link fence, and the scar is covered with it from one end to the other.

- Now cut two normal "I" tapes with rounded corners; their length depends on how big the scar taping has become. I call these large "I" tapes "fake anchors."

- Again, with these "I" tapes, tear the paper across the middle and remove it until just before the ends; stretch the first tape from the inside out with flat fingers, applying **very, very light stretch**.

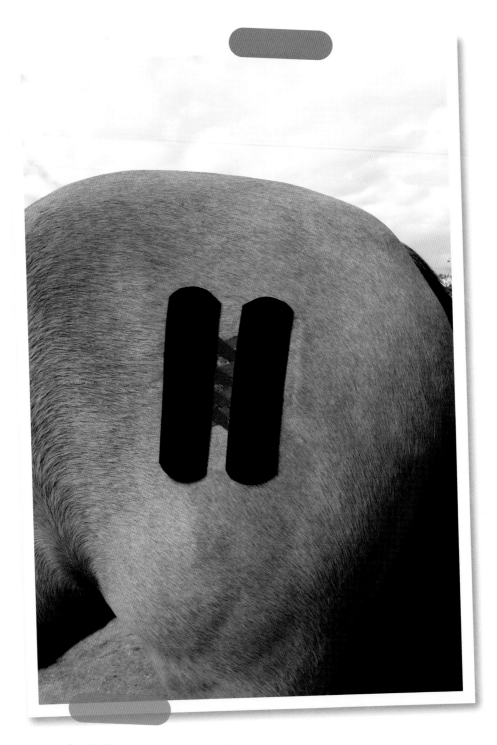

Fig. 17.6: The scar taping, now with its "fake anchors" applied, covering the ends of the "chain-link fence" of smaller tape strips completely.

- Apply this first "I" tape parallel to the scar, taping over one set of ends of the chain-link fence, covering the ends of the smaller tape strips completely.

- Apply the ends of the large "I" tape without any stretch, as usual.

- Apply the second large "I" tape the same way, covering the opposite ends of the smaller tape strips on the other side of the scar taping.

- Then gently rub over the entire finished application to activate the adhesive. Since there are so many small strips of tape involved, rub really carefully so you don't accidentally rub them right off.

These large "I" tapes applied parallel to the scar are not just anchors and protective layers to help keep the ends of the smaller strips of tape in place. The way they are applied—with minimal stretch, compared to the medium stretch you applied to the smaller strips—creates a different kind of stimulation for the skin. The scar tissue is stimulated by the smaller strips applied to it directly, but also by the interactions between the smaller strips and the additional layer of tape over them. That is why I call these larger strips "fake anchors"—real anchors have no effect at all on the taping application they are anchoring, but these strips are impacting the overall effectiveness of the scar taping by creating that additional stimulation parallel to the scar.

An Important Note for Scar Taping!

A scar treatment and the application of a scar taping should always take place only **after the wound has healed completely!**

This means:

- when the wound is completely closed from the outside;

- when any scabs have fallen off completely on their own;

- when any existing stitches have been removed.

The newer a scar is, the better your chances of success in treating it. But even a scar that is already several years old can still be treated effectively. It will just take longer to see results, because the connective tissue becomes less and less elastic over time.

Generally speaking, scar treatment and scar taping are never a one-time thing. This tissue is very tough and "stubborn," and therefore requires repeated treatments. Sometimes this can take months with older scars, during which the scar must be taped and massaged weekly.

Scar taping:

Direction of application: From the inside out, from the center of the scar outward.

Recoil: Toward the center of the tape strip, and thus the center of the scar.

Effect: Reduction of tension in the scar tissue, and stimulation of regeneration for inelastic and rigid connective tissue.

More Examples of Scar Taping

All of the following case studies and taping applications are *supportive* measures intended to complement veterinary, physiotherapeutic, or osteopathic treatments!

Scar Taping after Bone Chip Operation

After successful chip surgery on this horse's hock, a scar taping was applied along the scar. The stitches for the small incision had been removed by the vet the day before. The scar taping was secured at the top and bottom with "fake anchors." The application remained on the horse for three days and was then removed by the owner. The scar tape was then repeated six more times at weekly intervals.

Scar Taping for an Older Paddock Injury

This was an older injury in the shoulder area—the horse had been kicked while he was out in the paddock about two years ago, and had had a superficial skin injury that healed on its own. However, the scar tissue was extremely firm, which affected his movement, and especially his ability to reach forward with his foreleg.

Here is the scar taping I applied along his scar, with "fake anchors" above and below. I explained the application and demonstrated the process to the owner, and she independently repeated it at two-week intervals for six months. All this was combined with regular monthly scar treatment and massage.

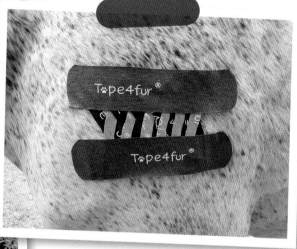

Fig. 17.8: A scar taping at the height of the shoulder blade after a paddock injury.

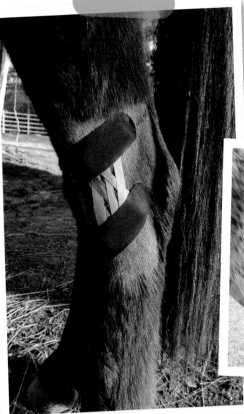

Fig. 17.7: A scar taping applied after bone chip surgery on the hock.

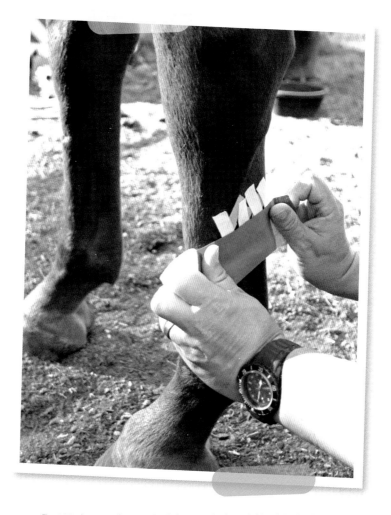

Fig. 17.9: A scar taping on a healed cut on the lateral side of the foreleg.

Scar Taping after Getting Caught on the Pasture Fence

This was a relatively fresh injury to the outside of this horse's foreleg—she had sustained a superficial laceration after getting caught on her pasture's fence. The wound was not sutured, and had healed on its own. However, the scar tissue was very firm and inelastic, and the fascia on the affected leg was also restricted. After loosening the fascia and massaging the scar, I applied a scar taping along the length of the scar with "fake anchors." The application was repeated every two weeks for two months, with the tape usually remaining on her leg for 4–5 days each time.

Chapter 18

Hoof Taping

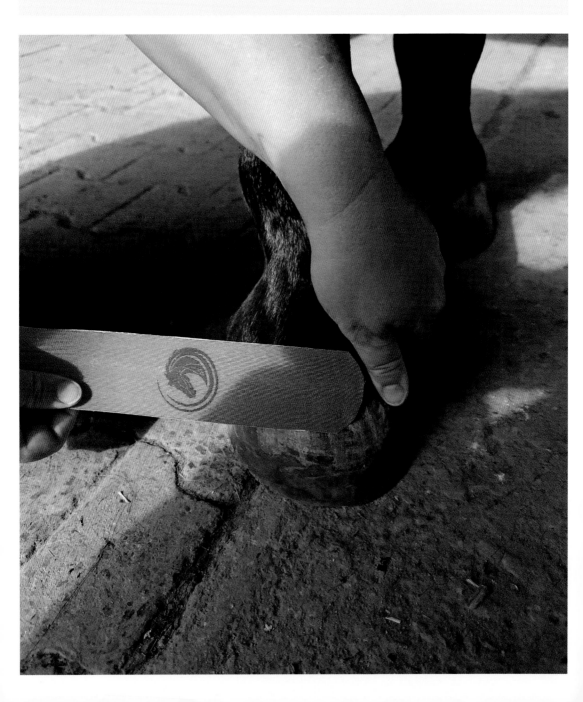

When Is a Hoof Taping Recommended?

Hoof taping is recommended in multiple situations—first and foremost, in cases of poor hoof quality. Since hoof cells are built in the coronet band, a taping application on the band can stimulate and positively influence the formation of hoof cells by increasing blood circulation and thus bringing more minerals, nutrients, and oxygen to the area. Increasing circulation in the area of the coronet band can also be very helpful for horses with extremely cold legs.

Furthermore, the area around the coronet band also contains a lot of sensory cells involved in body perception (proprioception), and you can use a hoof taping to facilitate and stimulate body awareness here—for example, with horses who consistently weight their hooves unevenly or incorrectly, or tend to shuffle with or drag their toes (provided you have already ruled out blockages or other issues in the leg as a cause).

How to Apply a Hoof Taping

You need a single "I" tape that is the right length to go once around the coronet band with the ends overlapping; the **end-to-end technique** is used.

- For very flatly angled hooves, it is helpful to have a helper hold the hoof up as if to pick it. For hooves that are not as flat, you can apply the tape while the horse is standing normally. The horse should stand on solid ground and not in sand, shavings, or straw.

- The hoof and coronet band must be clean and dry!

- Remove about an inch of the paper backing at one end of the tape strip, and apply this primary base without any stretch to the front of the hoof at the level of the coronet band, parallel to it. Approximately half of the tape should adhere to the hair above the coronet band, and the other half should be applied to the hoof wall.

- While gently pulling off the paper, apply the tape strip along the coronet band once around the hoof in the same way—with half of the tape applied to the hair and half to the hoof—using the 10 percent pre-stretch as it comes off the paper.

- The last inch of the tape strip is applied without stretch, as a secondary base.

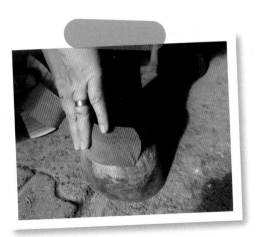

Fig. 18.1: Application of the primary base of a hoof taping.

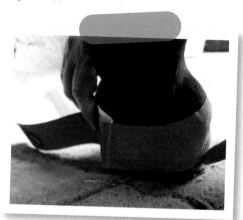

Fig. 18.2: Applying the hoof taping continuously along the coronet band.

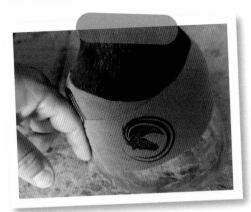

Fig. 18.3: Completed application of a hoof taping.

The ends can overlap by an inch.

- Rub vigorously but carefully over the tape strip to activate the adhesive.

Quick Tip: Any application where tape is adhering to the hoof will hold particularly well!

In general, it is easiest to always start on the front of the hoof with this hoof taping, as this is where you have the widest and most accessible contact surface. However, if you want to stimulate hoof cell growth, it is a lengthy process, and the application must be repeated again and again until the hoof has grown down all the way once. If you are applying the taping repeatedly like this, then the position of the primary base should be shifted from time to time, and applied at the inside of the leg and at the outside, too. Otherwise, the primary base will always be in the same place; since it is applied with no stretch, there is no recoil, and therefore not as much stimulation for the tissue beneath it. So in order to stimulate the hoof all the way around, it is a good idea to position the primary base in different places every now and then.

Hoof taping:
Direction of application: Once around the coronet band.
Recoil: Once around the coronet band.
Effect: Support of hoof cell growth, improvement of hoof quality; support of circulation; improvement of proprioception.

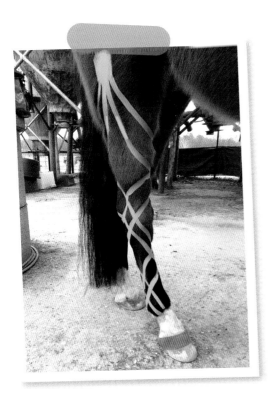

Fig. 18.4: A hoof taping combined with a proprioception taping.

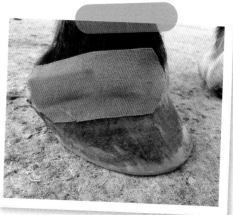

Fig. 18.5: Partial hoof taping.

More Examples of Hoof Taping

All of the following case studies and taping applications are *supportive* measures intended to complement veterinary, physiotherapeutic, or osteopathic treatments!

Hoof Taping in Combination with Proprioception Taping

Among other things, hoof taping stimulates body awareness and can therefore be combined very well with a proprioception taping of the same limb, if the entire limb is affected by an incorrect distribution of weight or limited proprioception. Proprioception taping is described in detail in chapter 20 (page 148).

Partial Hoof Taping to Stimulate Specific Points

If you believe in Traditional Chinese Medicine (TCM), and want to stimulate the end points of certain meridians—ting points—you can also apply a hoof taping that runs only part of the way around the coronet band. I taped this horse partially in order to stimulate the lateral ting points of his hind legs.

Chapter 19

Stifle Sling Taping

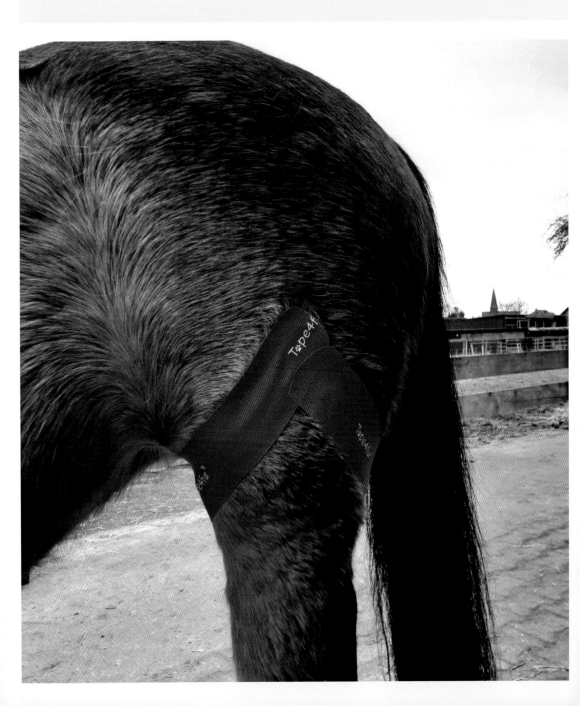

When to Apply a Stifle Sling Taping

More and more often, horses suffer from problems with the stifle and patella. Older horses, for example, commonly develop arthritis in the stifle. Younger horses often have problems with patella fixation, or, on the other hand, problems with weak stifle ligaments.

Unfortunately, due to the anatomical conformation of the horse, the stifle and patella can only be taped in a suboptimal way. You may want to consider the possibility of a stabilization taping as described in chapter 13 (page 98) to address instabilities in the joint.

It is particularly difficult to tape the patella in horses, because it is so deeply embedded in the flank and is not as easily accessible as it is in humans, where it rests on top of the knee and is easily palpable. Even in dogs, the patella is much easier to palpate and to tape than it is in horses, because in most breeds it is anatomically much freer.

But in cases of general muscular atrophy in the hindquarters, a stifle sling taping is worthwhile to give more support to the whole limb. It is best to combine this with appropriate muscle tapings. This application is also helpful in cases of ataxy and general instability of the hindquarters.

Be aware: On the inner thigh, the structure of the horse's hair is different, and the skin can be extremely oily. This can significantly compromise the stickiness of kinesiology tape. Therefore, this area should **always be rubbed down with baby powder beforehand and wiped clean with a microfiber cloth!**

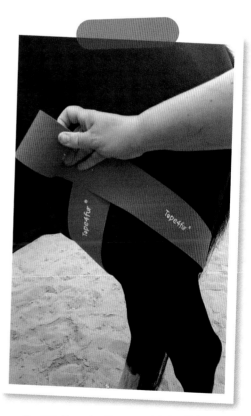

Fig. 19.1: Measuring the appropriate length for a stifle sling tape.

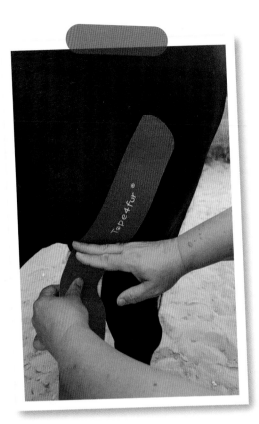

Fig. 19.2: Along the lateral side of the leg, the 10 percent pre-stretch of the tape is used for the stifle sling taping application.

How to Apply a Stifle Sling Taping

One long "I" tape with rounded corners is required for this taping, at the length necessary to allow it to pass once around the thigh (see fig. 19.1); the end-to-end technique is used.

- Position the tape roll against the outside of the leg, centered on the femur, and measure once around the stifle joint, horizontally along the inner thigh, around the popliteal fossa, and back to the starting point. Cut the tape with rounded corners.

- Remove approximately 2 inches of the paper backing from one end of

the tape strip, and apply this primary base without any stretch and with a back-up at the same starting point as for your measurement in the previous step. If you do it this way, the primary base is already going to be oriented forward and downward, pointing toward the stifle joint.

- Apply the first section of the "I" tape, using flat fingers and the stretch with which the tape comes off the paper (that 10 percent pre-stretch). Gently pull off the paper backing and apply the tape immediately until you reach the lateral side of the stifle joint.

- In the area of the joint gap, remove a little bit of the paper and apply the tape with moderate stretch until you reach the medial side of the stifle.

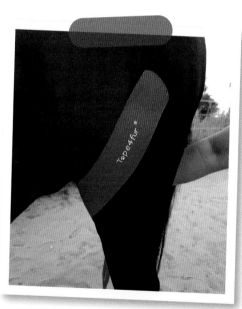

Fig. 19.3: Moderate stretch around the joint gap and the popliteal fossa.

Always make sure you are not holding the tape with pointed fingers.

- On the inside of the leg, apply the tape as it comes off the paper, horizontally along the inner side until you reach the popliteal fossa, again using the 10 percent pre-stretch of the tape.

- In the area of the back of the stifle, as before in the area of the joint gap, apply the tape with moderate stretch, up to the outside of the popliteal fossa.

- The remainder of the "I" tape is then applied with that 10 percent pre-stretch as it comes from the paper, going forward and upward toward the primary base.

- The secondary base is applied completely stretch-free, with a back-up.

- The secondary base should overlap with the primary base, thus forming a closed loop and providing optimal stabilization for the limb.

- Rub vigorously but carefully over the tape all the way around to activate the adhesive.

Stifle sling taping:
Direction of application: Going around the extremity with moderate stretch in the area of the joint gap and popliteal fossa.
Recoil: Multidirectional.
Effect: Supporting the stability of the leg, giving the leg an "upward lift."

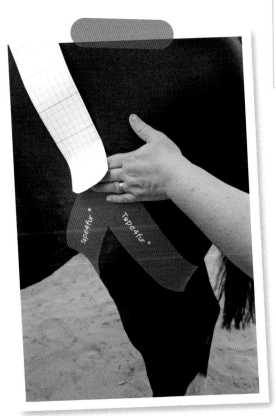

Fig. 19.4: The "I" tape is applied with its 10 percent pre-stretch, looping back to the initial starting point of the application.

More Examples of Stifle Sling Taping

All of the following case studies and taping applications are *supportive* measures intended to complement veterinary, physiotherapeutic, or osteopathic treatments! They can be used during rehabilitation as well as during training.

Stifle Sling with Activation of the Hind Leg Musculature

The stifle sling tape has no real variations, but it can be combined with other taping applications depending on the issue you want to address, as described at the beginning of this chapter.

This was an older German sport pony that was rather weak in the hindquarters; he had noticeably atrophied hind musculature. I combined a stifle sling taping with some muscle taping for the hamstrings and biceps femoris muscles, to support and stimulate muscle activity.

Stifle Sling Taping for Gait Instability

In cases of gait irregularity, uneven footfall, dragging hooves, frequent stumbling, or similar problems that are combined with instability in the stifle or hock, a stifle sling taping can be combined with a proprioception taping.

Any blockages or other physical issues must of course be ruled out beforehand. Lameness must be brought to the attention of a veterinarian!

The proprioception taping shown here will be discussed in detail in chapter 20 (page 148).

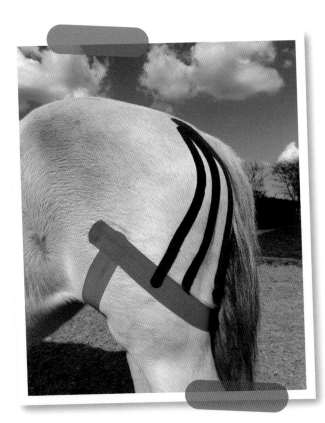

Fig. 19.5: A stifle sling taping combined with some muscle taping.

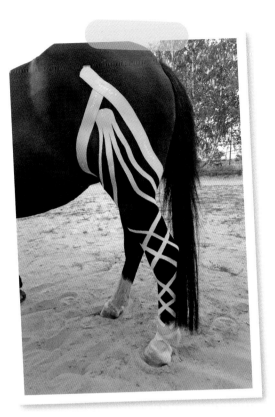

Fig. 19.6: A stifle sling taping in combination with a proprioception taping.

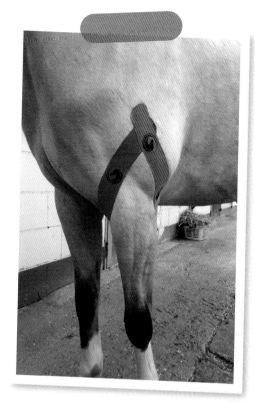

Fig. 19.7: A sling taping for the front leg and elbow.

Elbow Sling Taping

The sling taping can also be used on the forehand for problems such as elbow instabilities. These occur much less frequently than instabilities in the hindquarters and stifle, but they do happen. The procedure remains the same. Start on the outside of the leg, in the middle—at the level of the humerus—and then tape around the elbow gap with moderate stretch; continue horizontally along the inside of the leg and then use moderate stretch again underneath the point of the elbow; then bring the tape strip forward and upward and end on the outside of the leg again. Make sure you stay below the "crease" on the inner side of the leg so the tape does not rub off when the horse is walking.

Chapter 20

Proprioception Taping

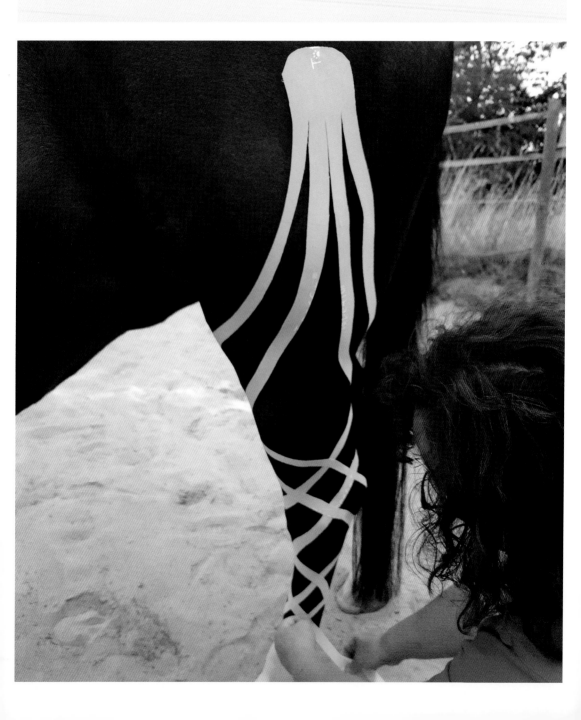

When to Use a Proprioception Taping

Proprioception was discussed at the beginning of the book in chapter 3 (see page 16). As a quick review of the basics: the term "proprioception" describes perception or awareness of the body and its position in space. This body perception can sometimes be impaired. In most cases, this manifests as uneven weighting of the limbs or an uneven gait pattern, even though there is no blockage or muscular impairment.

This kind of issue is often the result of a prolonged period of uneven posture, due to pain or blockages. Even after these causes are eliminated, an altered gait pattern or incorrect weighting has developed and become a habit over a longer period of time. The body has simply "gotten used" to the incorrect movement and perceives it as normal. To help correct this "misprogramming," a proprioception taping can be applied.

All taping applications—*all* of them— address body perception to some degree, because many proprioceptors (sensory cells that contribute to the sense of body perception) are located directly around the roots of the hair. But the proprioception taping is special in that it is applied without any stretch, and therefore has no recoil. Since you just want to stimulate the proprioceptive sensory cells, recoil in the tape is neither necessary nor desired.

The effect of a proprioception taping comes in the moment in which the horse moves with it applied. This creates very small shear forces between the tape, the hair, and the hair root, which in turn leads to stimulation of the proprioceptors—without affecting other sensory cells, such as mechanoreceptors for muscle activity.

This stimulates body perception in the affected limb or area, and consequently the movement process, and as a result, the affected joints and muscles are mobilized and activated.

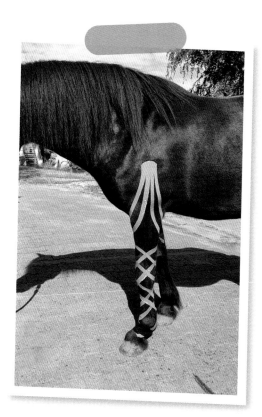

Fig. 20.1: Completed application of a proprioception taping on the front leg.

How to Apply a Proprioception Taping

For a proprioception taping for an entire limb, you need a fan tape with an even number of fingers (four fingers is optimal). On the forehand, measurements are taken from the level of the humerus, and on the hindquarters, from the level of the femur, all the way to the ground; then add about 8 inches to that length. The **end-to-end technique** is used **WITHOUT ANY STRETCH AT ALL** in the tape.

- Tear the paper backing across at the transition between the fingers and the base of the fan tape cut, and fold the edges over. This will make it easier to grasp these edges later.

- Remove the paper completely from the base, and apply it without any stretch and with a back-up, proximally at the level of the humerus, or the femur if you are applying this taping on the hindquarters.

- Start with one of the outer fingers; pull the paper off a section and hold the tape so that it only barely does not sag. Do not actively stretch the tape!

- In this unstretched state, apply the tape in a spiral pattern, working your way down around the entire leg toward the hoof. Remove a section of paper backing, take out the 10 percent pre-stretch in the tape, and then apply the tape without any stretch.

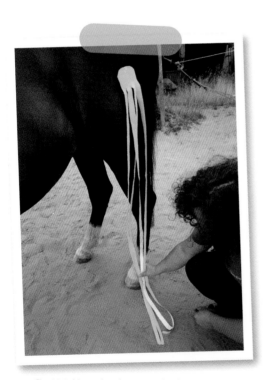

Fig. 20.2: Measuring the appropriate length of tape.

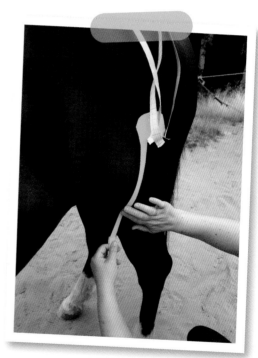

Fig. 20.3: Application of the first tape finger.

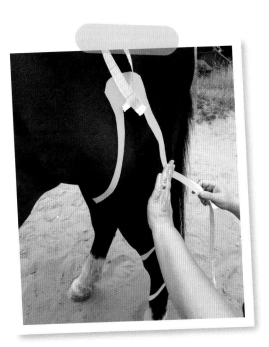

Fig. 20.4: Applying the second tape finger in the opposite direction from the first one.

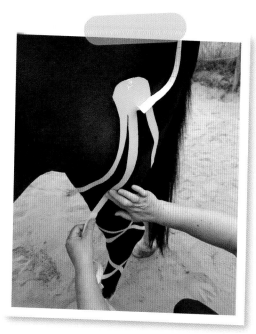

Fig. 20.5: The inner finger is applied parallel to the outer finger next to it, just a little bit lower.

- Next, take the opposite outer tape finger. Apply it using the same technique—without stretch, spiraling around the leg—but work your way around the leg in the opposite direction from the first tape finger.

- The two tape fingers should cross at several points on the leg, once they are both fully applied.

- Then apply the two inner tape fingers. The technique is always the same: apply without any stretch, in a spiral progressing downward toward the hoof.

- Each of the inner tape fingers is placed a little lower and applied parallel to the outer finger that is next to it, spiraling in the same direction as that outer finger.

- All four finger ends are also applied stretch-free, of course.

- It is a good idea to secure the thin finger ends with a stretch-free cross anchor so the tape fingers do not get caught in straw, shavings, or grass and detach prematurely.

- Carefully rub the tape fingers to activate the adhesive.

When this taping is complete, the limb is encased in the tape fingers, which cross each other in several places. The entire leg is thereby addressed and stimulated. It always looks a little bit like the horse is wearing "fishnet stockings"!

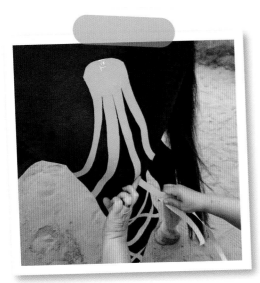

Fig. 20.6: Application of the last tape finger of the proprioception taping.

Proprioception taping:
Direction of application: Stretch-free, from proximal to distal, spiraling around the leg.
Recoil: No recoil, since there is no stretch anywhere in the application.
Effect: Stimulation of body perception; improvement of gait pattern and weight distribution due to shear forces between tape and skin during movement.

More Examples of Proprioception Taping

All of the following case studies and taping applications are *supportive* measures intended to complement veterinary, physiotherapeutic, or osteopathic treatments! You can use a proprioception taping in rehabilitation, but also specifically during training to address an affected limb or area more strongly.

Some examples of how to combine a proprioception taping with other applications can be found in chapter 18 (page 138) and chapter 19 (page 142).

Partial Proprioception Taping for the Lower Leg

If a movement restriction does not affect the entire limb, a partial proprioception taping can be applied to the lower leg to target this area more specifically. Here, for example, this horse's movement from the shoulder was even with her other side, but the situation changed from the carpal joint down. Any blockages must of course be ruled out or released beforehand. Here everything was also taped stretch-free.

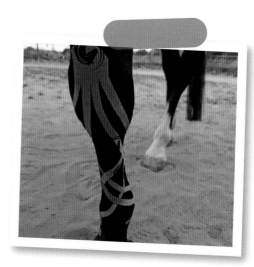

Fig. 20.7: A proprioception taping for the lower leg.

Partial Proprioception Taping for the Carpal Joint

If, for example, you only want to stimulate one joint, because there were previously blockages there that led to a restriction in movement, you can use a proprioception taping to target that joint by itself. Again, the joint should be enclosed as completely as possible. In this case, two fan tapes were used; I applied them medially and laterally to enclose the joint in this case. Even though it might look like a partial lymph tape for the carpal joint, it is not, since it is applied stretch-free.

The black cross tapes to either side were stretch-free anchors to prevent premature detachment, since the carpal joint has a relatively large range of motion when it flexes.

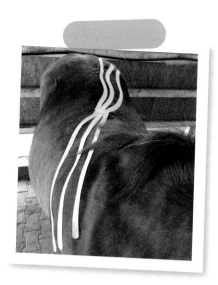

Fig. 20.9: A diagonal body proprioception taping.

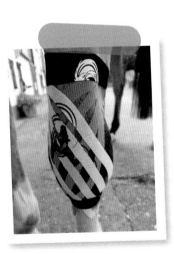

Fig. 20.8: A proprioception taping for the carpal joint.

Body Proprioception Taping to Prevent Diagonal Overloading of the Legs

In the same way we humans are right- or left-handed, and tend to have a preferred stance or starting foot, horses also have a preferred side, and are very diagonal in their loading pattern, which means they either load the "right fore to left hind" diagonal more or the "left fore to right hind" diagonal more. This is perfectly normal. But sometimes it can lead to overloading of one of these diagonals. In these cases, we can use a body proprioception taping to bring the horse's body awareness to his weaker diagonal.

Two very large fan tapes are needed for this taping. The base of the first fan is applied centrally on the back, and the fingers are then guided along the weaker diagonal toward the affected foreleg, without any stretch. The base of the second fan tape is taped centrally on the back, overlapping the base of the first fan tape, but the fingers of this fan tape are applied stretch-free along the weaker diagonal toward the affected hind leg.

If you want to use this application for training, then only use it for lungeing or ground work. Riding with it does not work well—due to the saddle's position and the rider's weight, the shear forces between the tape and the fur are limited, if not restricted, and the full effect of proprioception taping is lost.

Chapter 21

Corrective Posture Taping

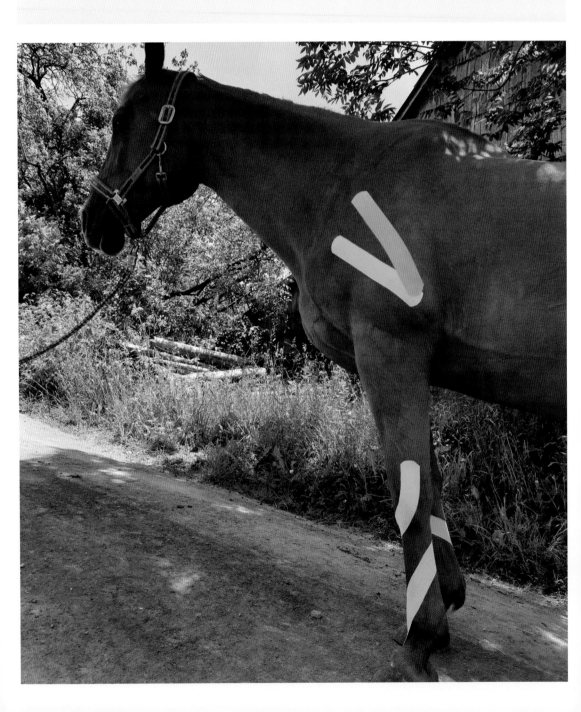

When to Use a Corrective Taping

The question of when to apply a corrective taping can be answered quickly and easily: Corrective taping is used for congenital or acquired abnormal positioning and postural issues. It doesn't matter whether the issue is a toe-in or toe-out stance, base-wide or base-narrow, internal rotation or external rotation of a limb, or, or, or....

Corrective taping primarily uses the recoil of the tape to guide a limb into the correct

position. That means this kind of taping is not necessarily based on anatomical principles such as the locations of muscles or tendons, but rather is primarily using the mechanical direction of the recoil of the kinesiology tape to compensate for incorrect positioning.

The most frequent cases I deal with in this regard are newborn foals that are born with a position issue of some kind. Since the tissues of foals are still very soft, it's usually possible to achieve good results very quickly. But corrective taping applications can also be used to help older horses that have become accustomed to an abnormal body position over the years. In these cases, the application must be repeated more often over a longer period of time in order to sustainably "reprogram" the bad posture away. And with older horses, the whole process has to be supported with a lot of bodywork, since the body's structures have to be mobile enough to "follow" the guidance provided by a corrective taping.

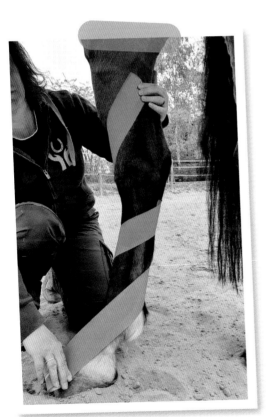

Fig. 21.1: Measuring the required length of tape strip for an outside rotation from the hip out, using the right hind leg.

How to Apply a Corrective Taping for External Rotation of a Limb

For this taping application, you need one "I" tape that is rounded at both ends. The length varies considerably depending on the issue you are addressing and the length of the leg, as can be seen both here and in the following examples. The **end-to-end technique** is always used, with mild to moderate stretch, and there is one simple rule to follow: **always tape toward the position issue!** As already described in chapter 8 (page 44) in the explanation of the end-to-end technique, the recoil always runs opposite the actual direction of application—toward the primary base, and, in this case, that means in the direction of the correct position.

In the following step-by-step example, we

are dealing with an acquired abnormal position of the hind leg, starting at the hip joint with an external rotation of the whole leg. Thus, the application starts near the body, on the inside of the leg, and the taping direction follows the external rotation; the recoil forces will then stimulate the limb in the other direction, back to a straighter position.

The inside of the upper leg should be rubbed down with baby powder and a microfiber cloth before you start taping.

- Completely remove the paper backing from the first 2 inches of the "I" tape, and apply the primary base—without any stretch—centrally on the inside of the leg, just below the stifle. The base thus already points in the direction of the external rotation.

- Hold the tape with flat fingers and apply it diagonally forwards and downwards, following the external rotation in a spiral around the leg, with moderate stretch.

- Tape several times around the leg. This creates a stronger impulse to correct the position than if the tape is applied around the limb only once.

- Apply the end of the tape strip, the secondary base, without any stretch, as always.

- Rub vigorously but carefully over the tape strip to activate the adhesive.

- If necessary, secure the application at both ends with stretch-free cross anchors.

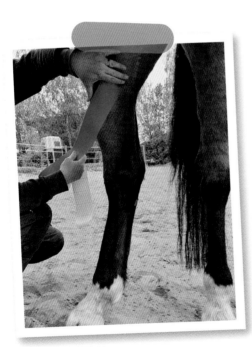

Fig. 21.2: When you are addressing an external rotation of the leg, the primary base is applied medially, on the inside of the leg.

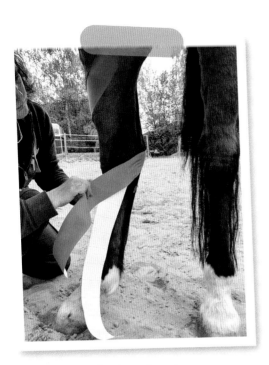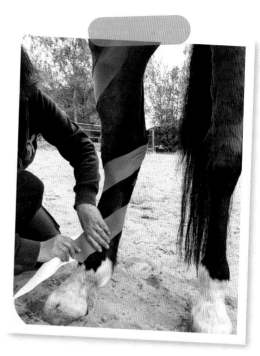

Figs. 21.3 and 21.4: In cases of abnormal positioning of the whole limb, apply the corrective taping with moderate stretch, and spiral around the leg several times.

With adult horses, I always use moderate stretch when applying a corrective taping. With foals, however, where everything is still so soft and not fully formed, mild stretch or even the stretch with which the tape comes off the paper backing—that 10 percent pre-stretch—is usually enough. In addition, foals usually do not need additional work done besides the taping. They react much faster to the stimulation of the tape than older horses.

In cases of acquired abnormal positions that have had years to turn into habit, the simultaneous physiotherapeutic treatment of the surrounding structures is very important.

Among other things, the horse's muscles will have adjusted to the incorrect position over time, and are much less likely to find their way back to the desired position without the help of massage and stretching.

OBSERVE: There are less than five minutes between figs. 21.3 and 21.5, and the horse has not been manually repositioned by anyone. He has corrected himself on his own, with the stimulation of the corrective taping. Observe the external rotation of the hind leg at the start of the taping in fig. 21.3, and the position of the limb five minutes after taping is completed in fig. 21.5.

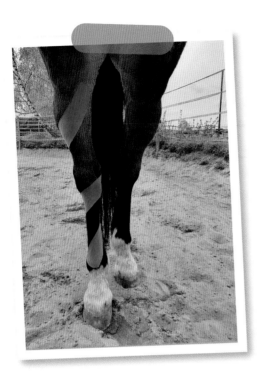

Fig. 21.5: Completed application of a corrective taping, with the leg already in a much better stance.

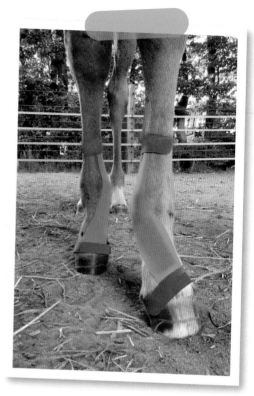

Fig. 21.6: A corrective taping for toe-wide posture.

Corrective taping:

Direction of application: Toward or following the abnormal position.

Recoil: Toward the correct position.

Effect: Bringing limbs with acquired and congenital position issues into the physiologically correct position.

As described at the beginning of this chapter, a one-time application of a corrective taping is not enough. The application needs several repetitions in order to have a lasting effect.

More Examples of Corrective Taping

All of the following case studies and taping applications are *supportive* measures intended to complement veterinary, physiotherapeutic, or osteopathic treatments!

Toes Wide

This foal was born with a mildly toe-wide posture, with slight external rotation from the fetlock down. I positioned the application so that it started medially on the cannon bone on both sides. I then taped over the front side of the fetlock with mild stretch, and continued laterally toward the outside of the hoof. The

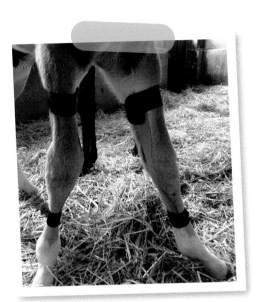

Fig. 21.7: Corrective taping for "knock-kneed" carpal joints and base-wide toes.

An X-ray confirmed abnormal positioning of 18 degrees between the lower carpal row and the cannon bone of the right foreleg of this horse, with weak muscle tone in the limb. As a result, the horse had a base-wide stance from the carpal joint down.

I applied a tape strip medially, from proximal down toward the abnormal positioning (unfortunately not visible due to the angle of the photograph) with the recoil directed proximally, to help bring the elongated medial structures into a straighter position. The shortened structures on the opposite, lateral side of the leg were taped with compensatory tape from distal at the fetlock up to proximal just below the elbow. These corrective tapes were secured with multiple cross anchors. The application was repeated twice a week for four weeks.

Quick Tip: The hair of foals is often greasy, probably to help keep them warm—but it makes getting the tape to stick more difficult. Rub down the target area with baby powder and a microfiber cloth before taping it, and the tape will adhere better.

tape was secured with cross anchors at the top and bottom. I explained the application to the owner, and she repeated it multiple times over a few weeks.

For a toe-in stance, the application would be applied in the opposite direction—from the lateral side of the leg toward the medial side of the hoof.

Base-Wide and "Knock-Kneed" in the Forelegs

This foal had a good muscle tone, but stood very wide on the ground, and his carpal joints were slightly "knock-kneed." I applied a tape strip on the inside of each leg from proximal to distal, toward the position issue, with mild stretch, and then secured the applications with cross anchors proximally and distally. This was shown to the owner, and she repeated it independently several times. After about four weeks, there was hardly any sign of the issue anymore.

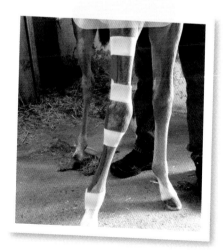

Fig. 21.8: Corrective taping for abnormal positioning in the carpal joint.

Chapter 22

Crosstapes

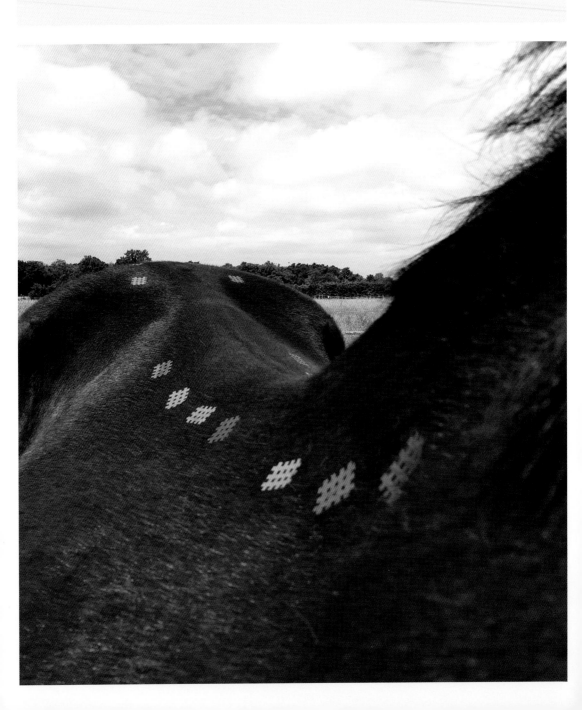

What Are Crosstapes, and How Do They Work?

Grid tapes, also called crosstapes, are made of cotton, but unlike kinesiology tape, the fabric is actually a cotton-silk mixture. They do not have any spandex fibers, either, and therefore are not stretchable at all. However, these little waffle-shaped tape patches are coated with acrylic adhesive, and are completely medication-free. Crosstapes are available in different sizes and colors. The main distinction between crosstapes and kinesiology tape, along with the lack of stretch in crosstapes, lies in the fact that crosstapes are statically charged—or rather they become statically charged when you pull them off their plastic carrier foil.

The surface of the skin and hair of horses (and humans) has a certain static charge of its own. Where there is disease, or a change or disturbance in the tissue underneath, and thus a change in the acid-based tissue environment, this static charge can change in the affected areas. The special shape of crosstapes does have a slight "lifting effect" on tissue, but their more important purpose is to restore that static charge to normal, stimulating energy flow and supporting pain relief.

Crosstapes can be combined with kinesiology tape or used separately. They are used for special treatment of small areas and are often used for trigger points, stress points, and pain points. Therapists who believe in the principles of Traditional Chinese Medicine (TCM) often use them on acupuncture points, for additional support of acupressure, acupuncture, or laser acupuncture. They can also be used on scars, and on small animals, in instances where even 1-inch-wide kinesiology tape would be too big.

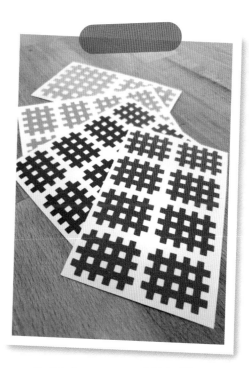

Fig. 22.1: Crosstapes are available in different sizes and colors.

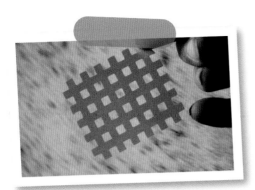

Fig. 22.2: In order to avoid altering their static charge, crosstapes should be handled very carefully.

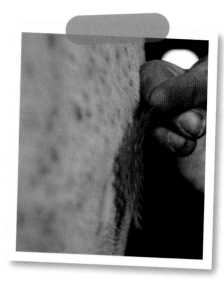

Fig. 22.3: Slide the crosstape carefully over the hair; it will adhere to the affected area by itself.

How to Handle Crosstapes

- Carefully lift one corner of the crosstape from the plastic foil with your fingertips, or with **plastic** tweezers, and then gently peel the entire crosstape off.

- Hold the crosstape only at this one corner, and then carefully slide it very close to the hair over the affected area.

- Due to the change in the static charge of the hair and the charge of the crosstape itself, the crosstape will find the affected area on its own and pull itself to the hair at the affected point, adhering there firmly.

- **DO NOT RUB OVER THE CROSS-TAPE.** You might accidentally rub it off again—and friction is not desirable in this case anyway, as it would alter the static charge of the crosstape.

Crosstapes, like kinesiology tape, can remain on the hair as long as they will stick. They fall off by themselves when they have done their "job." It is a good idea to carefully brush around the affected area when grooming the horse, while the crosstape is on

More Examples Using Crosstapes

All of the following case studies and taping applications are *supportive* measures intended to complement veterinary, physiotherapeutic, or osteopathic treatments!

Acupuncture Points

In addition to acupuncture, acupressure, or laser acupuncture treatments, a crosstape can be applied to the treated acupuncture point for additional prolonged support afterwards. The crosstape will remain in place until it falls off on its own. This crosstape is applied to the point Pericardium 9, which in TCM practice is treated for problems of the hoof, among other things.

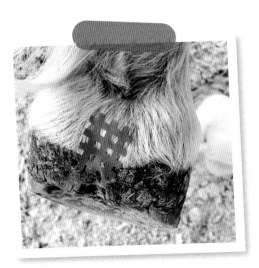

Fig. 22.4: Stimulation of the acupuncture point Pericardium 9, according to TCM.

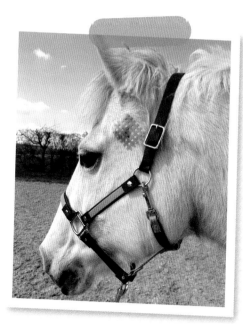

Fig. 22.5: Treatment of the TMJ with a crosstape.

Temporomandibular Joint (TMJ)

As a follow-up treatment after the release of temporomandibular joint blockages, you can apply a small decompression taping on the joint (see chapter 12, page 90) or you can apply a crosstape to stimulate circulation again. After dental treatments, when a horse has worn a mouth gate for an extended period of time, it is also a good idea to apply a crosstape to the TMJ. They can be placed on one side or on both sides, depending on whether both sides need to be addressed.

Scars

Crosstapes can also be used to support scar treatments. You can apply a scar taping, as described in chapter 17 (page 130), or you can use several small crosstapes along the length of the scar. In most scars, the skin's static charge and energy flow are disturbed, and crosstapes help correct this issue. Just as with an actual scar taping, the entire scar should be covered with the crosstapes.

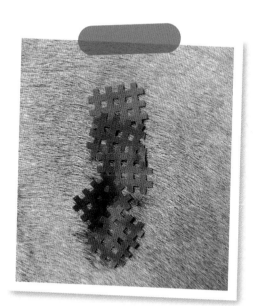

Fig. 22.6: Multiple crosstapes along the length of a scar.

Acknowledgments

As always, my biggest thanks go to my husband, who supports me fully in all my projects. Though his actual job is in the IT field, he is now also an absolute taping expert.

I would also like to thank Martha Cook from Trafalgar Square Books, who already supported me through the US publication of the first edition of *Kinesiology Taping for Horses*, as well as *Kinesiology Taping for Dogs*, and who was interested in continuing that partnership with this new edition.

Along with all the horses that have modeled here in the book, I would like to specifically thank Tonga and Balou. Tonga is our cover model this time, and my own horse Balou has modeled so many times that I have lost count. Also, my great thanks to the horses Chaya and Sophie for being such patient taping models. Thanks to all my equine patients, for always letting me treat and tape you with such patience—so much that some of them unexpectedly became models in this book as well.

And of course I would also like to thank all the horse owners who entrust me with their animals for treatment, especially the horse owners whose animals have made it into this book. Thank you, dear Steffi, for providing your Tonga as a model for the cover photo.

I also have to say thanks to my Canadian colleague Christa Veinotte, CEO and owner of Hestaband, for immediately picking up on the chance to support me with this book by providing her Hestaband products as well.

References

Akupunktur und Phytotherapie beim Pferd [Acupuncture and Phytotherapy for Horses], Carola Krokowski, Sonntag Verlag, Stuttgart 2010

Muskelatlas des Pferdes für Physiotherapeuten [Atlas of the Horse's Muscles for Physiotherapists], Katja Gühring, Senden 2012

Veterinary Anatomy of Domestic Animals, Horst-Erich König and Hans-Georg Liebich, Thieme, 2020

About the Author

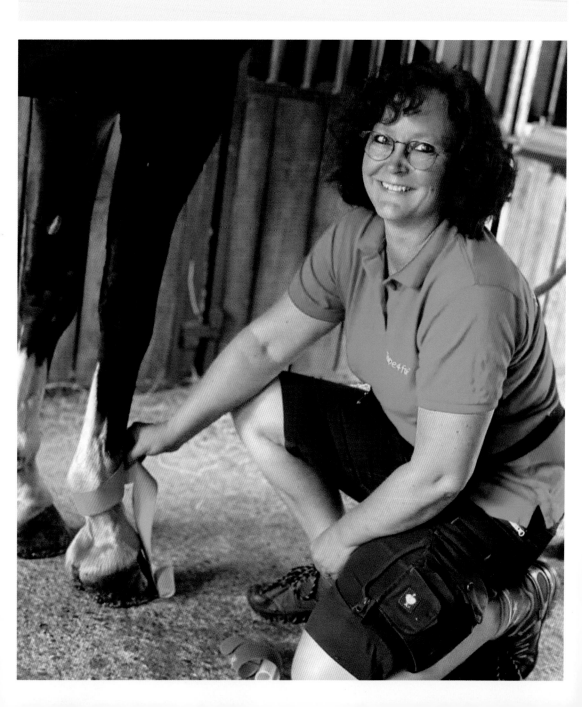

Like so many of my colleagues, my own horse brought animal physiotherapy to my attention many years ago. A problem that the vet couldn't fix was then solved by an animal physiotherapist, and the process fascinated me so much that I said to myself, "What that woman can do, I want to be able to do, too!"

During my training as an animal physiotherapist, I also took a course on "Flexible Taping for Horses" at the same time, because I wanted to know what these colorful adhesive tapes were all about.

From the beginning, I was enthusiastic about what could be achieved with kinesiology tape, and through a stay of several years in the USA, and contact with the management of a local tape company that developed a tape for horses there, my taping knowledge deepened even more.

During my daily work as an equine physiotherapist, I was asked again and again what taping was all about, and since I was able to explain it well enough to make myself understood, the call for a book and courses quickly became loud, and one thing led to another.

I gave my first taping courses during my time in the USA (today, I focus on Germany, Austria, and Switzerland), and then in the fall of 2016, the first edition of *Kinesiologisches Pferdetaping* was published in German by Müller Rüschlikon Verlag. The first English edition of *Kinesiology Taping for Horses* was published in 2018 by Trafalgar Square Books.

For six years, I have been the German and European distributor for the aforementioned American taping company. And then a deeply personal project for me went live in 2022, and, with 10 years of my own taping experience and help from fellow German animal physiotherapists, I developed my very own kinesiology tape for animals: Tape4Fur®.

Through a long testing and evaluating phase, we took care to develop a tape suitable for all types of animals, with all their various kinds of hair and fur. This tape has been tested with and successfully applied to horses, cows, goats, donkeys, dogs, cats, guinea pigs, bunnies, and many more furry friends.

Contact information:
If you have any questions about kinesiology taping for animals, feel free to check out my website and social media, or email me directly.

www.horse-wellness.com
info@horse-wellness.com

https://www.facebook.com/katjashorsewellness
https://www.instagram.com/katjashorsewellness

You can also use our shop contact information:

www.tape4fur.com
info@tape4fur.com

https://www.facebook.com/tape4fur
https://www.instagram.com/tape_4_fur

Where to get kinesiology tape:
In Europe: www.tape4fur.com
In Canada: www.hestaband.com
Both brands also ship worldwide!